DR. JOE'S MAN DIET

LOSE 15-20 POUNDS, DROP BAD CHOLESTEROL 20% AND WATCH YOUR BLOOD SUGAR FREE-FALL IN 12 WEEKS

JOSEPH FEUERSTEIN, MD, ASSISTANT CLINICAL PROFESSOR OF MEDICINE, COLUMBIA UNIVERSITY

WITH GAVIN PRITCHARD, REGISTERED DIETICIAN, CERTIFIED EXECUTIVE CHEF

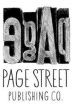

PAGE STREET
PUBLISHING CO.

PAGE STREET
PUBLISHING CO.

First published in 2016 by

Page Street Publishing Co.

27 Congress Street, Suite 103

Salem, MA 01970

www.pagestreetpublishing.com

Distributed by Macmillan, sales in Canada by The Canadian Manda Group.

19   18   17   16   1   2   3   4   5

ISBN-13: 978-1-62414-179-9

ISBN-10: 1-62414-179-X

Library of Congress Control Number: 2015909752

Cover and book design by Page Street Publishing Co.

Photography by Ken Goodman

Printed and bound in China

THIS BOOK IS DEDICATED TO OUR FAMILIES, PATIENTS
AND READERS, AND TO THE MEMORY OF ERIC LEVY, MD.

— "BROTHERS IN HEALING FOREVER" —

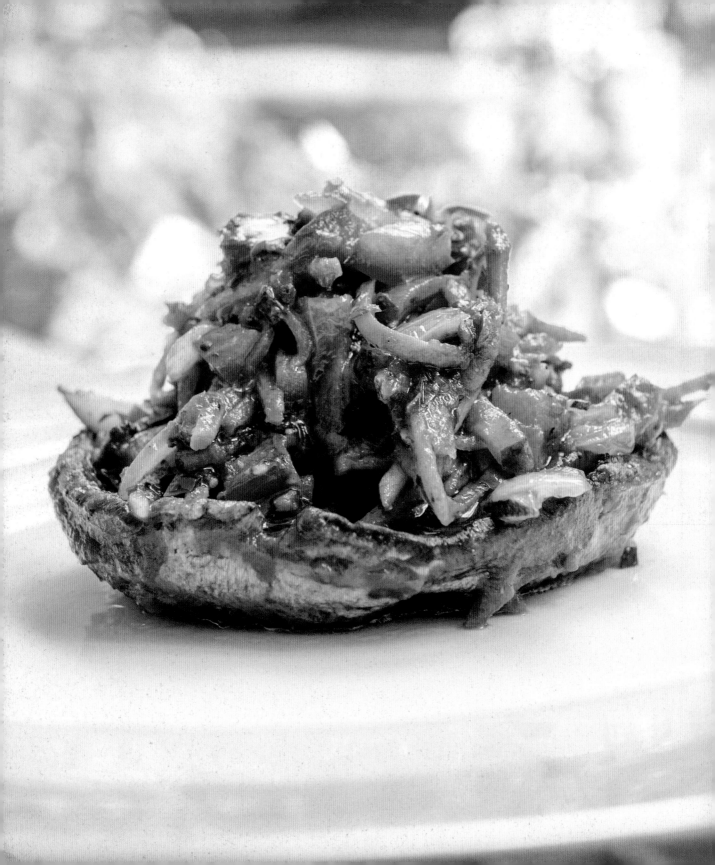

INTRODUCTION | 6

1

JUST THE FACTS | 8

SIMPLE AND NOT GOOD

2

BLOOD TESTS AND HORMONES | 28

GETTING ALL THE FACTS

3

THE "MONEY" | 52

WHAT EXACTLY TO EAT AND WHY

4

THE RECIPES | 64

5

HELPFUL HINTS | 174

AND HOW TO KEEP YOUR NEW BODY

ACKNOWLEGMENTS | 197
ABOUT THE AUTHORS | 198
REFERENCES | 199
INDEX | 204

INTRODUCTION

Dude, do you remember the good old days when you could eat pizza all day and still look slim and toned? When going to the beach was a joy, not an embarrassment because of your belly fat? Maybe you've seen your physician and been told to lose weight because your blood sugar, or glucose, is up and so are your cholesterol numbers.

Sound familiar? If this is you, you're not alone. There are millions and millions of men like you, not only in the United States but now all over the world.

Unluckily for you, you probably have metabolic syndrome: excess weight, high blood glucose, high blood pressure, and your blood tests show your cholesterol numbers are heading the wrong way. This is not good news because your risk of heart disease and cancer is increasing, which means your chance of dying prematurely is also increasing. I assume this is not your plan for right now.

So what do you do about it?

You might go to see your friendly neighborhood doctor, a very reasonable thing to do, and chances are the doctor will recommend that you improve your diet and start some form of exercise.

Sounds promising; sounds like you have hopes of a thinner, healthier future. Cool.

The only problem with that plan is that you're not sure exactly what is a good diet or what type of exercise is right for you. The devil is in the details, and there just aren't enough of them.

So you try something on your own with resolve and lots of enthusiasm but, unfortunately, lifestyle change is difficult and things go downhill fast.

Perhaps in three months you'll recheck your labs and see that the situation still has not improved. Your doctor is now offering you a prescription medication that you will be taking for the rest of your life!

Dude! The situation is bad.

If this describes you, you are not alone. The most recent research for the Centers for Disease Control and Prevention states that 71 million Americans over the age of 20 have elevated cholesterol, and the number is rising.

So what is wrong with taking a small, white pill every day for the rest of your life? For some people the answer is: nothing. But there are many others who just don't fancy being dependent on a pill for the rest of their lives to keep them from having a heart attack.

I get it.

And for those people who think that they can just medicate their way to happiness and health, I have some bad news.

In April 2014, researchers from the University of Tokyo published the results of a 10-year, 28,000-person study that showed that people who started taking cholesterol-lowering medication (like Lipitor, Zocor, Crestor and the rest of the gang) started eating more and gaining more weight, compared to the people not on these drugs.

Now from the outset, let me be very clear about two things: first, I don't believe for a second that the medications cause increases in appetite and weight gain; and second, statin medications are lifesaving for the right patients.

The point, my friends, is that this study clearly shows that people who want to rely on small, white pills do just that—they take the pills and continue to eat whatever they wish with reckless abandon. So they put on weight, and pretty soon their cholesterol isn't the only thing they have to contend with. Now they have blood glucose issues, gout and high blood pressure, and one simple pill becomes a whole pillbox.

I see guys like this every day. I've literally seen tens of thousands of people for weight, cholesterol and blood glucose issues over the past seven years.

So if you find yourself overweight with troubling lab test results, I know exactly what you need. This is not my first rodeo, and unlike almost all other diet books ever written, my eating plan is proven to work, based on two published clinical studies.

Again, this is all I do for a living, so I can tell you what will work and what won't—with all the details you will need for a total lifestyle makeover that includes an eating plan that is not so difficult that you won't enjoy eating anymore.

What you are about to read is exactly what I have told the last 10,000 people I have seen like you.

The book is divided into five chapters.

Chapter 1 describes how metabolic syndrome is bad for you, along with all the other facts you should know to get you motivated to get with the program.

Chapter 2 talks about all the important lab tests, so you'll really know what is going on before the journey begins. I also go over all the various hormones that can help or hinder you in your quest to find your mojo again.

Chapter 3 is the actual eating plan—simply written, used 10,000 times and has worked like a charm, always.

Chapter 4 contains approximately 60 recipes to give you some idea of the variety of dishes you can eat. As my wife, four kids, three dogs, two cats and fish will all assure you, I cannot cook anything that is remotely edible. You will therefore be pleased to know that these are not my recipes but those of my incredibly talented colleague, Gavin Pritchard, who combines his encyclopedic knowledge of nutrition as a practicing registered clinical dietician with his flair for and love of cooking (he is a trained chef). Gavin's easy-to-follow recipes are going to inspire both you and anyone else you decide to buddy up with for this lifestyle challenge. He'll show you that life doesn't end on the day you start a diet!

Chapter 5 gives helpful hints that will keep you going, including specific details on the other vital things like exercise, sleep and stress reduction that you will need for the new you.

This program takes 12 weeks, and by the end of this period, you should have lost 20 pounds (9 kg) and watched your blood glucose, cholesterol and pants size plummet. You will sleep better, have more energy and start to feel your mojo the way you did when you were toned and 20!

Like every other doctor, I am a scientist, so I promise you two things:

– Every statement I make is based on solid scientific evidence, and at the end of the book, I have included an extensive reference section so that you can check out the details.
– In an effort not to completely bore you, I am going to talk only about the details of a few scientific studies in each chapter.

Let's get started, then.

JUST THE FACTS

SIMPLE AND NOT GOOD

Here is the problem, in a nutshell, cramped and crowded: being obese isn't just a problem of appearance and self-esteem. Obesity will kill you, just as an elevated level of the wrong type of cholesterol or blood glucose will. It won't happen immediately. But there is a mass of scientific research showing that it will get you in the end.

Not convinced? Let me show you the latest evidence to prove my point. And to do it, instead of citing 50 studies that all say the same thing, I am going to describe just one study, because one is all you need.

A study was published in November 2013, looking at more than 4,000 people in San Antonio, Texas, over a seven-year period to see what their risk of developing heart disease (the number one killer in the USA) or diabetes was, if they were thin or fat or if they had metabolic syndrome.

The results are pretty depressing, as expected.

The risk of developing diabetes doubled for those who were obese (we will talk about what that actually means in Chapter 2) compared to those who weren't, and the risk of heart disease increased by 40 percent.

The kicker is that, even those whose cholesterol panel was good and whose blood sugar, or glucose, was not elevated (so they didn't have all the features of metabolic syndrome, they were just fat), still had an increased risk of developing diabetes and heart disease. In other words, just being heavy is enough to speed you to an early death.

The other finding of this study is even more sobering. It turns out that, even if you are thin, the risk of developing heart disease is nearly triple, and the risk of diabetes skyrockets by 250 percent if you are thin and have bad labs.

The take-home message is that either metabolic syndrome (being fat on the inside) or obesity (being fat on the outside) significantly increases your risk of getting diabetes (which causes blindness, kidney failure, nerve pain, amputations and all manner of other health woes) and heart disease (which causes death).

I'm not being subtle, but this whole situation is not very nice, so there is no time for subtlety.

Now let's move to a little science to help me show you what the underlying problem is: that what you eat may be causing your early demise. But first, I'll begin with a question.

Do you have a pet peeve? Are there certain things that unsuspecting friends and colleagues do that really get under your skin?

I am sure I have many, but one of my professional pet peeves is this: When my patients return to me after four weeks of eating better, feeling thinner, healthier and more vital, and happily report to me that they haven't eaten any carbs for the last four weeks. I know it sounds ridiculous, but when people refer to my diet as another low-carb diet (à la Atkins or South Beach), I get annoyed. I therefore correct them by saying, "You are still eating lots of carbs. There are plenty of carbohydrates in your fruit, vegetables, low-fat dairy and in the special grains I instructed you to eat (you'll hear all about this very soon, I promise). What you have cut out is all that extra sucrose, starch and saturated fat that you weren't using and didn't need."

You see, the basic philosophy behind my eating plan is not to entirely eliminate a whole food group, as seen in low-carbohydrate or low-fat diets. My approach helps you reduce just certain types of carbohydrates and fats, namely sucrose, starches and saturated fats that are slowly killing you.

What is so bad about sucrose, starch and saturated fat? Why are they the enemy?

To answer that question, permit me to take on each of my opponents, one at a time.

SUCROSE TABLE SUGAR: SWEET, ADDICTIVE AND DESTRUCTIVE

Table sugar is a type of carbohydrate, and like all carbs it is made of carbon, hydrogen and oxygen, three of the most important substances on the planet.

You may recall from school that there are actually different types of carbohydrates which are classified depending upon the number of sugar molecules they contain (see picture below). There are single sugar molecules like glucose (the stuff that floats around in your bloodstream) and the sugar found in fruit called fructose. Then there are types of carbohydrate made up of two sugar molecules like the bad boy sucrose (the white stuff we use to powder donuts, aka table sugar) and lactose (the sugar that makes milk taste sweet). Starches and fiber are made up of lots of sugar molecules.

TYPES OF CARBOHYDRATES	CARBOHYDRATE MOLECULES
GLUCOSE AND FRUCTOSE (FRUIT SUGAR) MOLECULE	
SUCROSE (TABLE SUGAR) AND LACTOSE (MILK SUGAR) MOLECULES	
STARCH AND FIBER MOLECULES	

So here is a question for you: What is the difference between our friendly fiber and our nemesis starch?

If you look at the diagram above, they appear exactly the same! The answer is that we can't digest fiber, so it bulks up our stool and is passed out the other end. Starches, on the other hand, can easily be digested, and they are broken down in our gut into their individual glucose molecules, then they head straight into our bloodstream, increasing our blood glucose and making us sick.

So why is this all so important?

In a few pages you'll learn all about starch and why it is making you ill, but for now, let's focus on sucrose and see how that makes us feel.

At the risk of stating the obvious, sucrose is one of the main constituents of some really bad foods: soda (a whopping 35 grams of sucrose in every single fizzy can!), fruit drinks, candy, cookies, ice cream, desserts and so on.

Junk is made of sucrose. Sucrose is therefore junk. And it will kill you.

In February 2014, the Centers for Disease Control in Atlanta published a huge study that looked at the diets and health of more than 30,000 people over a 15-year period. They found that people who got more than 10 percent of their total daily calories from sucrose are 30 percent more likely to die of heart disease than people who obtained less than 10 percent of their calories from that sweet, sticky substance.

You may be wondering if the other sugars like fructose or lactose are just as lethal. The answer is that it depends on whether you are eating the whole food or an unnatural and unholy concentrated version of the thing. Here is what I mean:

In August 2013, a large study from Harvard University's School of Public Health was published online in the *British Medical Journal*. The study analyzed data from over 187,000 nurses and doctors, looking at their patients' diets and risk of developing diabetes. The results are remarkable. Those who ate lots of apples, grapes and berries, even though these fruits are full of fructose, reduced their risk of developing diabetes by up to 26 percent. Those who drank fruit juice, however, increased their risk of developing diabetes by 8 percent. The authors of the study explained that the significant variation in diabetes risk is probably because of the increased fiber content and antioxidants found in whole fruit.

Putting it plain and simple, eating a whole apple means that you aren't just eating fructose; you are also consuming a fiber called pectin at the same time. If, however, you decide to juice your way to good health, you'll throw away all that great fiber found in the pulp and be left with just the sugar water to consume, pushing you further along the way to eventual diabetes.

The take-home message is **juice = sugar = junk**. That being said, if you want to purchase a food blender and eat the entire fruit (pulp and all) blended into a smoothie, be my guest; you are just saving your teeth the trouble of chewing.

Now that you have a basic understanding of the different types of sugars, let me show you the hidden sugars that are not listed on nutrition labels.

Food labels list the amount of carbohydrates in each serving size. On the next page is the nutrition label of the all-powerful Twinkie to help illustrate this key point.

NUTRITION FACTS	
CALORIES 150 (627 KJ)	
TOTAL FAT	4.5 g
SAT. FAT	2.5 g
TRANS FAT	0 g
CHOLESTEROL	20 mg
SODIUM	220 mg
TOTAL CARBS	27 g
DIETARY FIBER	0 g
SUGARS	19 g
PROTEIN	1 g
CALCIUM	20 mg

A Twinkie contains 27 grams of carbohydrates, which is a lot. It has 19 grams of sugar—mostly sucrose, and it has 0 grams of fiber. Hmmm, if it has a total of 27 grams of carbohydrates, but only 19 grams of it is sugar, then there are an extra 8 grams of carbohydrate that are neither sugar nor fiber (27-19 = 8). These are the hidden sugars that are found in starch.

What do I mean by that?

We just saw the chemical structure of sucrose and starch. Sucrose is made up of two glucose molecules, and starches are composed of many glucose molecules. Clearly, sucrose and starch are not the same thing. But starches start breaking down into sugars the moment they reach your mouth, making starch essentially the same as sugar. Even so, starch doesn't have to be listed as sugar on the nutrition label.

Most people who read the Twinkie nutrition label look at just the amount of sugars listed. They may say to themselves that it has only 19 grams of sugar, which isn't too bad. But the truth is that the entire 27 grams of carbohydrate listed on the label are either already sugar or are about to become sugar. If you add those extra hidden sugars, the snack becomes a little less appealing. Reading labels is important because if you just look at the sugar content listed on the side of the box, you'll miss the masses of hidden sugars that the manufacturer doesn't have to declare.

STARCH: TOO MUCH OF A GOOD THING

Just to remind you, starch is made up of lots of individual glucose molecules.

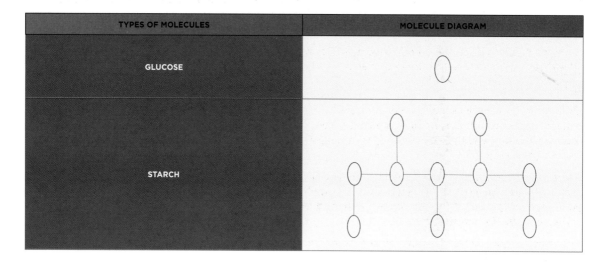

TYPES OF MOLECULES	MOLECULE DIAGRAM
GLUCOSE	
STARCH	

Again, the kicker here is that the instant you put any starch in your mouth, enzymes in your saliva break it down to the sugar it was originally made of. You can therefore see why I often say to patients that starch and sugar are basically the same thing.

Now let's look at the history of starch and human nutrition, so we can start to understand how everybody got to be so fat and unhealthy.

Up until 10,000 years ago, humans were not eating grains at all. Our ancestors were eating lean meat, poultry, nuts, seeds, fruit, vegetables and fish. They were also not eating any dairy products as they hadn't yet domesticated cattle. If this eating approach sounds familiar, it is the basic approach of the Paleo diet that everybody raves about. I've seen this diet work well in clinical practice, and I like the authenticity of the approach, but most patients find it too hard to keep because it restricts too many things, for example, no grains at all, not even the good ones. The zero-grain approach I see with my Paleo-patients makes them feel hungry a lot of the time because grains temporarily give us the feeling of being full (satiety).

Now being hungry in the era of Paleolithic humans was probably to be expected, and this grainless hunger was a significant motivator for early humans to spend most of their daylight hours hunting and foraging for food. However, this same hunger today can present a challenge if you are confined to a desk all day with only a 30-minute lunch-break. Therefore, although the Paleo plan is one way to go, my advice is to stick to my plan instead; you'll still end up healthy but with less hungry resentment! Since those bygone days of spears, sweat and the savannah, people on every continent of the globe have learned about agriculture and now eat the staples of the world: bread, rice, potatoes, pasta, corn and maize. What is common to all these foods is that they are high in calories, most of which come from starch.

I have a theory why the world moved from the Paleolithic days of constant snacking to the modern convention of three solid meals a day earned by the "sweat of thine brow." As Paleolithic people realized when they began tilling the fields during the Neolitihic Era, it would be fairly inconvenient and not very economical to leave work every two hours to forage for berries and nuts. A better plan would be to consume a calorically dense and glucose-laden food in the morning that would keep the engine running till lunch.

By enjoying a similar starch-filled repast for our midday meal, we could all push through till sunset and our evening sustenance. And that, my friends, is how we all got turned on to starch.

Now don't get me wrong, even today if you are a day laborer or field hand and are working all day harvesting grains or chopping wood, as many of our forefathers did for most of their lives, then you better eat something packed with calories, like whole grain bread, brown rice, sweet potatoes, al dente pasta, corn or maize.

But what happens if you don't work in manual labor but spend nine hours a day sitting behind a desk? Would you still need to eat all the extra starch found in your lunch sandwich or your pasta salad with shrimp?

Clearly not.

Unfortunately, most of us are still brought up with the idea that a balanced meal is meat, two veggies and a starch. Although this diet worked when people were very active throughout the day, nowadays we are all mostly sedentary, and this way of eating is no longer appropriate for our lack of movement, leading to health issues and obesity.

Remember, your body is still designed to hunt and gather, but you aren't running around all day trying to skewer things with a spear. The only hunting and gathering you are likely to do is while standing in front of your open refrigerator at the end of the day, hunting for something sweet on the top shelf and gathering something salty from the bottom one.

Even the U.S. government's recommendations for a healthy diet don't consider the new reality that most of the population is now sedentary.

The U.S. Department of Agriculture's (USDA) MyPlate recommends that 55 to 60 percent of calories should come from carbohydrates, particularly whole grains. The problem with this is that it assumes that we are still all very active and will therefore easily be able to burn off the thousand or so carbohydrate calories in our everyday activities.

Again, if you are a manual laborer or can exercise for an hour every day as the Institute of Medicine recommends, then this 200–300 grams of carbohydrate, which is predominantly in the form of starch, will be easily used, and the USDA's guideline is very good dietary advice.

But for the rest of us, all that excess fuel we eat but don't use up is converted by our bodies into fat for storage, as our bodies wait for the famine that never arrives.

So how does all that extra starch we didn't need but ate anyway, because that was how we were brought up, turn into fat? The answer is simple. It is all courtesy of insulin, the body's hormone that is designed to store every excess calorie by turning it into fat.

Insulin is produced in the pancreas and helps maintain normal glucose levels in the bloodstream by making the glucose in your blood enter other tissues of your body. Insulin is therefore released by your body when your blood glucose level rises to get the glucose out of your bloodstream and bring your blood glucose levels back down into the normal range.

So where does all that sweet sugar go after leaving the blood? It goes into the liver, muscle and, most importantly, fat cells, where it will be converted into fat by a process called lipogenesis.

And, yes, you did hear me correctly. The extra sugar that you got from that last candy that you didn't need will be entering your waiting fat cells and instantaneously turned into fat. All thanks to our storage hormone—insulin. Why does this happen, you may be asking yourself. The reason is simple: Humans are built to hunt and gather through plentiful and sparse seasons, through sun and snow. Your body still hasn't realized that you now have a constant and reliable food supply. It still thinks that it should save every extra ounce of energy for the famine that never comes.

While we are on the subject of insulin, one important side note that you should certainly be aware of is that when your blood glucose levels are high, your body will make large amounts of insulin. This is true especially if your cells become sluggish or less responsive to the effects of insulin, a condition called insulin resistance. Now, remember that insulin is the storage hormone working to conserve all the excess calories as fat. If your blood insulin levels are elevated, you'll have a harder time losing weight.

Luckily, every day I see that the eating plan you'll be meeting soon will drop your insulin levels back to normal in those 12 weeks, quick and easy, for sure!

So if starch is just lots of glucose molecules packed together, it isn't hard to see how eating too much starch could increase your blood glucose level.

But how does too much starch cause an increase in our cholesterol? Again, our friend insulin is to blame. Here is how:

You eat a bag of potato chips. These deep-fried delicacies are packed full of starch, which is immediately broken down in your mouth into glucose. The glucose then floods into your bloodstream and your blood glucose levels start to rise. Your ever-vigilant pancreas senses the increase in your blood glucose and immediately releases insulin into your bloodstream, which will then allow all that glucose to enter the various tissues of your body and be used as fuel.

Much of the glucose is taken up by the liver and converted to a storage substance called glycogen.

Sounds good so far. But what happens if you eat a lot of starch and the liver stores of glycogen are already full? What happens to all that extra glucose that is still pouring into the liver cells?

These poor cells have no choice but to turn the glucose into fatty acids, which are then packaged together with special transporter proteins and released into the bloodstream as very low density lipoprotein (VLDL) cholesterol.

Simply put, starch breaks down into sugar, which eventually becomes cholesterol. Who knew that a potato chip could be so deadly!

You may think I am exaggerating? Let's look at the evidence.

On June 23, 2011, the *New England Journal of Medicine* published the combined results of a study that involved more than 120,000 people over a 20-year period. They concluded that the lowly potato chip was the number-one culprit for causing a gradual increase in weight over time. In fact, roughly half of the average 3.35 pounds (1.5 kg) a healthy, nonobese American gains over a four-year period can be caused by eating just one extra serving of potato chips every day.

Not a potato chip fan? How about some white rice with stir-fried chicken and vegetables?

White rice is another food packed with starch, which is quickly broken down by the body into glucose and therefore can cause your blood glucose levels to spike soon after you have eaten it. By the way, the speed with which a carbohydrate is broken down into glucose and causes an increase in blood glucose levels is known as its glycemic index (GI), and we shall learn all about this important concept below. First, however, let's finish showing you just how bad starchy white rice is for your body if you are sedentary.

The dietary composition of 40,000 men and 158,000 women from three large population studies was analyzed by researchers from Harvard's T.H. Chan School of Public Health. The shocking results showed that having more than five servings of white rice per week was associated with a 17 percent increase in developing type 2 diabetes.

I should state that the same study also showed a reduction in the risk of developing diabetes if people substituted whole grain rice for white rice. I am a firm believer that whole grains, yams, plantains, quinoa, buckwheat and couscous (that weird-looking stuff they sell at health food stores), which contain lots of starch, are much healthier for you than the useless white starches currently lining most of our pantries.

However, unless your weight is normal, your cholesterol and sugar are at a healthy level and your physical activity is daily and involves a fair amount of sweat, I would steer clear of these healthier foods too. You just can't afford the extra starch and calories just yet.

As I tell all my patients when I first put them on this eating plan, this is not a forever diet; this is a program to help get you back to how nature intended you to be, lean and active.

So far, we have established that too much sugar and starch is bad for you. They make us fat, they make our sugar and cholesterol levels go up and they also raise our insulin levels.

Let's recap and learn about the magic number.

- Junk food is packed with masses of sucrose. Junk food is lethal (what a shocker!) and therefore so is sucrose.
- The unnecessary and excess consumption of the starch-packed food staples of the world—bread, rice, pasta, potatoes, corn, maize and so on—by sedentary people is making everybody sicker as we speak.

Okay, so what about the magic number?

I can think of a lot of magic numbers, but in the world of weight loss à la *Highlander,* "there can be only one." 750. That, my friends, is roughly the number of calories you need to cut per day to achieve reasonable weight loss. And it doesn't matter if you cut fat (a low-fat diet as proposed by the American Heart Association) or you cut carbs (à la Atkins and South Beach). If you want to drop weight, you need to reduce your intake by 750 calories per day.

And just in case you are wondering how I came up with this magic number—I didn't. About four years ago, a large study was published in the *New England Journal of Medicine* comparing low-fat to high-fat diets and low-carb to high-carb diets. The bottom line of this study is that, in order to lose weight, it really doesn't matter what the composition of the diet is. What is important is that you cut approximately 750 calories from your diet per day. In other words, whether you cut carbs or cut fat doesn't matter as far as weight loss is concerned; it is all about the number of calories you cut.

But weight loss isn't the only thing we are interested in, I hope. How about dropping cholesterol and sugar levels and dodging the medication bullet?

The same *New England Journal* study also looked at drops in cholesterol levels in people on low-carb or low-fat diets. The study found that neither of the diets achieved a larger drop in the bad cholesterol, low density lipoprotein (LDL), than about 5 percent at the end of the two years.

At the end of this section I'll show you the data from my two published clinical trials that dropped the bad cholesterol by over 20 percent in only three months. I found that the types of food you eat when you are trying to cut calories, not just the amounts, is also important. Cutting back on certain food groups like starch, sugar and saturated fats will affect your blood glucose and your cholesterol levels in addition to your waistline.

As we need to cut 750 calories per day from our diet to achieve weight loss, perhaps now you can begin to see the simple logic of my diet:

- Cutting down on the starch-filled staples of the world (bread, rice, potatoes, corn, maize and so on) and sugar (candy, cookies, cake juice, soda) will cut out at least 600–700 calories per day from our plate and will therefore lead to significant weight loss.
- Getting rid of starch and sugar, the two great evils, will help reduce our insulin levels and drop our blood glucose and cholesterol to boot!

Again, the enemy is sugar and starch, not the entire carbohydrate food group. My diet is not a low-carb fest; it is a low-sugar and -starch fest!

There are plenty of carbohydrates in my diet, as you will see in detail in the next chapter. But none of the carbohydrates I encourage you to eat cause sudden and extreme increases in your blood glucose and insulin levels. All the carbohydrates you'll eat are low on the glycemic index.

You see, not all carbohydrates are created equally when it comes to insulin release and blood glucose levels. Sucrose, for example, has a high GI and so within 15 to 30 minutes of eating a spoonful of sugar, you'll see a rapid rise in your blood glucose levels. An apple, on the other hand, though it is also packed with carbs, causes a slow and gentle increase in your blood glucose levels because it contains lots of fiber, which slows down the rate at which the sugar in the apple is absorbed from your gut into your bloodstream.

But what is wrong with a diet that restricts your carbohydrate intake to 20 grams as opposed to the government-recommended 300 grams per day?

I am sure you know people who initially lost weight on low-carb diets like Atkins or South Beach Phase 1. You may have even tried one yourself. What is so bad about a low-carb diet?

The answer is that our bodies need to consume a certain amount of carbohydrates every day in order for our brains to continue to run on their favorite fuel—glucose.

The reason many dieticians and other health care professionals don't like the popular low-carb diets is that these diets include a daily carbohydrate intake that is so low that people on them are unable to maintain a constant supply of glucose to the brain.

What does the brain use for energy if it is glucose starved?

The brain will be forced to use substances called ketone bodies as its fuel. Ketone bodies are made by the body from our fat stores. A low-carb diet causes the body to break down its fat stores in order to feed the brain with ketone bodies. Breaking down fat means that you'll lose weight. Sounds great!

The problem is that ketone bodies are also potent diuretics—they make you pee a lot. As we humans are composed of nearly 50 percent water, a significant proportion of the initial weight loss you'll see on a low-carb diet is due to water loss. That's fine if you want to lose 10 pounds (4.5 kg) in 10 days for your daughter's wedding, but as it is water weight after all, it will come splashing back again if you stop your low-carb kick.

As I said before, with my diet we use the GI to choose other, healthier carbohydrates that still feed our brains with glucose but do not at the same time cause havoc with our blood glucose and blood insulin levels.

Now to our third archnemesis.

SATURATED FATS: THE C-GRADE OPTION

Saturated fats, killing you slowly with every bite! I'll start by explaining what fat is and why some forms of fat are bad news. We will also review some of the healthier fat options that are the main sources of fat in my diet, look at the evidence from the very low-fat Ornish diet and talk about some of the problems I have seen in clinical practice with this difficult way of eating.

Over the last 30 years, the conventional wisdom in Western medicine has been that lowering your fat intake will lower your weight and cholesterol. It is based on the fact that of the three major food groups, or macronutrients to use the scientific term, fats have twice as many calories as protein or carbohydrates do. Therefore, if you lower your fat intake you will obviously lower the total amount of calories you are eating every day, and you'll lose weight.

There is no doubt that this works. But first, let's look at what fats are, and then decide whether all fats are the enemy or whether it is a little more subtle than that, with only some types of fat being the enemy, while others may actually be our friends.

All fats are made up of three chains of fatty acids that are each separately attached to a backbone structure called glycerol.

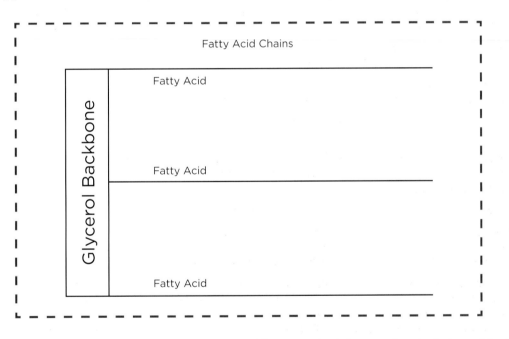

If the above structure passed you in the street, you wouldn't recognize it, but you do actually know it by its more common name. Ladies and gentlemen, the structure above that looks like a deformed letter E is, in fact, a triglyceride. Yes, that weird thing your doctor keeps on talking about that isn't cholesterol and whose levels seems to be getting ever higher in your blood whenever it's checked.

Triglycerides are little balloons of fat that are wafting around in your bloodstream. Their levels increase when you eat too much sugar and starch. That's right, your sugar and starch intake will not just increase your waistline and blood glucose, it will also raise your triglycerides. Now you see why sugar and starch really are the enemy.

But we still haven't worked out who our other opponent is, so back to the description of the different types of fat, and perhaps we will finally identify our foe.

In the diagram above, we were introduced to the term fatty acids. These are composed of chains of carbon and hydrogen atoms. We can classify our fatty acids as saturated, monounsaturated and polyunsaturated, depending upon the number of double bonds between the carbon atoms.

I am not going to bore you to death by showing the chemical structure of the different types of fatty acids, but I am going to tell you the reason it is important.

The chemical structure of saturated fats allows the fats to stack themselves in a closely packed arrangement and are solid at room temperature. Butter is a great example of a food that is solid at room temperature and packed with saturated fats.

Mono- and polyunsaturated fats have more double bonds in their structure so they can't pack themselves quite as nicely as their saturated fat cousins. They are therefore found as oils at room temperature. Fish oil and olive oil are two good examples of polyunsaturated fats.

Now we have met the whole family. Which one is the black sheep? Come on people, you know the answer to this one: it is the saturated fat.

To illustrate the point, let me quote the first line of an article that appeared in one of England's premier medical journals *The Lancet* in 1992: "In most countries, high intake of saturated fat is positively related to high mortality from coronary heart disease."

In other words, eating butter, cheese, steak and other delicacies that are laden with saturated fat increases your risk of having a heart attack. Or will it? That's right, I am questioning whether saturated fat is a real evil or just more of an annoyance.

You see, many in the alternative medicine world feel that the body needs saturated fat. According to some in the alternative medicine world, as long as you keep the number of calories coming from saturated fat at less than 10 percent of your total calorie intake per day, then eat away! And there is some evidence for this argument.

In 2010, the *American Journal of Clinical Nutrition* published a study of over 347,000 people who were studied for between 5 and 23 years. After analyzing the results the study concluded that "there is no significant evidence for concluding that dietary saturated fat is associated with an increased risk of heart disease."

In fact, a February 2015 paper by Scottish researchers published in the cardiology journal *Open Heart* went so far as to criticize the 1970–1980-era national recommendations to cut saturated fat intake in the United States and the United Kingdom, stating, "It seems incomprehensible that dietary advice was introduced for 220 million Americans and 56 million UK citizens given the contrary results from a small number of unhealthy men." In the same article, they also noted that the government's suggestion to replace fatty foods with carbohydrates (i.e., starches) "was probably not helpful and probably harmful to many."

So where are we now? What I often say to my patients is this: the two great evils, starch and sugar, are useless foods if you want to lose weight and improve your numbers.

Saturated fat isn't completely useless; it isn't a big evil, it's just a little one, but as there are much healthier types of fat that you could eat instead, I recommend emphasizing those instead.

Dr. Dean Ornish's high-fiber, low-fat, vegetarian diet has decades of research behind it that clearly shows his approach lowers weight and can even reverse heart disease. The Ornish diet emphasizes beans, fruit, vegetables and grains and avoids meats, nuts, seeds, full-fat dairy, alcohol, sugars like high-fructose corn syrup, and high-fat processed food.

He recommends that, of your total daily calories, only 10 percent should come from fat. Most people eat double or triple that amount. (And don't worry; my eating plan is laden with fat, the good types coming from nuts, seeds, avocado and olive oils!)

But the Ornish approach isn't just about food. It also includes 30 minutes of moderate exercise daily along with stress management techniques such as yoga, meditation and massage.

There is no doubt in my mind that the Ornish program works. I saw its results with my own eyes when the hospital in which I work ran an Ornish program for 60 of its employees. People lost weight and became physically fit for the first times in their lives. Their stress levels went down as their dress and belt sizes diminished.

The problem I eventually saw with the Ornish participants was that, after the program ended, people returned to their former habits, and their weight returned, along with their medications and inactivity. It is very hard to maintain this restrictive diet over the long term, and you have to be devoted to the cause.

Many people try a less extreme approach with fat than that employed by Dean Ornish. They carefully and diligently choose the low-fat options at every meal in the expectation that this will lead them to the nirvana of skinniness and better health.

I see patients like this every day and I invariably inform them of two important facts about low-fat diets. The first is that the low-fat option is usually high in carbohydrate instead. This is because if you can't have the smooth and comforting sensations of fat rolling around inside your mouth, then you will certainly settle for a sweet taste titillating your taste buds!

The second thing I explain to them is that not all fats are bad. We shouldn't try to do without an entire food group. I encourage people to switch their fat calories from butter and beef (saturated fat) to nuts, seeds and olive oil (mono- and polyunsaturated fats). All fats are not bad. In fact, a 1997 study in the *New England Journal of Medicine* that analyzed the diets of 80,000 women between the ages of 34 and 59 showed that replacing 5 percent of daily calories from saturated fat with unsaturated fats reduced the risk of heart disease by 42 percent! They concluded that replacing saturated fat with mono- and polyunsaturated fats was more effective in preventing heart disease than reducing overall fat intake. In other words, replace the bad fats with good fats; don't just throw out the baby with the bath water.

You'll soon see that my diet has some similarities to the Ornish plan, by emphasizing fruits and vegetables. However, where we clearly part ways is in the high consumption of starchy grains that he advocates and I strongly denounce; and in the mono- and polyunsaturated fats that he eliminates and I encourage.

I hope I have explained who our enemies really are and why the eating plan you will start isn't simply low in all fat or all carbohydrates but rather is reduced in only certain carbohydrates like sugar and starches and has less of certain fats like the saturated ones. This diet is therefore much more tolerable as it doesn't try to eliminate an entire family of food. Instead, we pick the good members of each family and avoid those bad cousins who wreak havoc and mayhem at every family function.

THE SCIENCE BEHIND IT ALL

I am going to go over the details of the 41-person and the 85-person published studies upon which this book is based. I'll be showing you a table that illustrates the key findings from the first paper: a 21-percent drop in bad cholesterol (a reduction comparable to that seen by taking prescription medication), a 12-point drop in fasting sugar, and an average weight loss of seven pounds (3.2 kg) over a period of four months. The key findings for the much more comprehensive second study were again a 20-percent drop in bad cholesterol, a glycated hemoglobin (a measure of blood glucose) drop from the brutally diabetic level of 7.5 percent to 6.5 percent (that is a better result than many diabetic medications have), a statistically significant drop in both systolic and diastolic blood pressure of 5 mmHg and a 14-pound (6.4-kg) weight loss over a 10-week period.

I am then going to compare my study's findings to those seen in the study on the Atkins, Mediterranean, the Paleo Plan and low-fat diets, and talk a little about those eating plans too. We will also look at the most recent study on the famous Weight Watchers program and compare their results to mine. We'll finish off this section with a brisk stroll through vegetarianism, plant-based whole-food diets, the theory behind the blood-type diet, gluten-free living and, at the very end of the section, I'll show you the study with results comparable to mine but with an eating plan that is much less fun to be on.

That all sounds terrific, Joe, but why should I care about comparing the results of different studies to each other? Why should I care about this science stuff anyway?

You may be thinking in the back of your mind: If my diet works, it works; if it doesn't, it doesn't; enough already with the science! I don't disagree with that approach. I freely admit that I want you to keep to my diet because it works for you, not because it has been proven to work in a clinical study. So, again, why should you care about all this science?

The reason is simple: many of the fad diets that are unveiled to the general public have undergone no clinical studies before their grand debut that would show whether they are safe or even work, a recurrent complaint that I hear from my physician colleagues all the time.

For example, in 2008, a study that compared a low-fat to an Atkins to a Mediterranean diet over a two-year period was published in the prestigious *New England Journal of Medicine*. We shall look at the results of this seminal study in a few pages, but for now I just want to point out that this large study was undertaken years after the original Atkins diet first came out in print.

Hippocrates, the father of modern medicine, advises that we should let our food be our medicine. Never were truer words spoken, in my opinion. Food is medicine. Food can do many of the things that pharmaceutical medications do, and then some.

The Food and Drug Administration does not allow prescription medications to just appear on the shelves of your local drug store without having undergone years of clinical studies of their effects on both animals and humans. So if food is medicine, then wouldn't you like to know that a new dietary approach has already had some scientific research done on it, showing that it is both safe and effective?

I know that I would, and I also truly believe that you deserve to know that this diet is both safe and effective too. It is for this reason that I spent three and a half years of my life undertaking two clinical studies that you will now read about.

A few years ago I worked as an integrative family physician at a private office in Greenwich, Connecticut. For a number of years I had been using the dietary approach that this book is based upon with all my overweight patients, and had noticed that they seemed to be losing weight, lowering their cholesterol and reducing their fasting sugar levels whenever they adopted these simple dietary changes. Science is about observation, so I decided to look at the charts of the patients I had seen who had weight issues, cholesterol or high blood glucose levels during the calendar year 2009. I contacted the Institutional Review Board of Greenwich Hospital and obtained permission to undertake this patient chart review. Then the real work began on this, my first study.

I looked at 243 of my patients' charts and was able to use the results from 41 of the patients. You are probably wondering why over 80 percent of patients were unable to be included in the study. Let me assure you that it wasn't because they didn't lose weight or see their labs improve. In fact, almost every patient's health improved in some way while being on this diet. The reason most of the patients could not be part of the study is that they were already taking cholesterol-lowering or sugar-lowering medicine that had been prescribed by their other physicians. I was looking for people who weren't on any cholesterol or sugar medicine so that we could see if this diet really worked without the need to factor in the effect of those medicines.

Of the 41 patients who tried my diet, 28 (68 percent) of them were able to stick with it. This is a pretty high number, proving that a low-starch, -sucrose and -saturated fat diet is not as difficult a diet as you may have thought it would be. The other 13 (32 percent) patients who were in the study couldn't handle the diet and went back to their bad old habits. We shall see what happened to them in due course.

I bet you probably think that the patients who succeeded must have been superhuman beings who could control their every urge and could probably move objects with their minds. Not so!

The average person was in his or her mid-50s, overweight, and there were slightly more men than women. You see, this first study showed that this eating plan is a Man Diet because it works best for men.

And that, my fellow brothers, is something that I have seen every day for the last seven years that I have worked as a consulting physician in integrative medicine.

It isn't that women don't do great. I assure you that this eating plan will work for your wives, mothers, sisters and daughters, but the most striking results in terms of speed of weight loss and dramatic lab value improvements is with the guys, plain and simple. And the guys in the study and the guys I see every day in my office are just like you! Not one is a secret demigod with powers to help him control himself. Just plain, simple men who have let themselves go and want to get back to the way they used to be. And if you keep to the plan and are a good marine, that is precisely what will happen. Guaranteed. Now, back to the study.

I looked at the laboratory results of all the patients before they started the diet and then looked at their repeat laboratory test after they had been on their new eating program for between four and six months. The table below (which comes straight out of the published study) shows you the before and after results of the two groups. To remind you again, 70 percent of the people stuck to the diet (the compliant group) and 30 percent of the people just couldn't (the noncompliant group).

COMPLIANT				NON COMPLIANT		
VARIABLE	COMPLIANT GROUP—BEFORE THE DIET	COMPLIANT GROUP—AFTER 6 MONTHS ON THE DIET	COMPLIANT GROUP'S AVERAGE CHANGE DUE TO THE DIET	NONCOMPLIANT GROUP—BEFORE THE DIET	NONCOMPLIANT GROUP—AFTER 6 MONTHS	NONCOMPLIANT GROUP—AVERAGE CHANGE
WEIGHT (LBS, KG)	179.5 (81 kg)	172.5 (78 kg)	- 7 (-3 kg)	188.3 (85 kg)	190.3 (86 kg)	+ 2 (+1 kg)
BLOOD PRESSURE (MMHG)	125/78	117/75	- 8/3	133/85	136/87	+ 3/2
TOTAL CHOLESTEROL MG/DL	242	189	- 53	226	250	+ 24
BAD LDL MG/DL	158	115	- 43	151	166	+ 15
GOOD HDL MG/DL	56	52	- 4	54	58	+ 4
TRIGLYCERIDE MG/DL	133	111	- 22	105	134	+ 29
FASTING GLUCOSE MG/DL	104	96	- 8	91	96	+ 5

I am sure that some of you don't like tables as it brings back memories of fifth grade math, braces and crushes. I get it. So to highlight the take-home message, I will give you some key bullet points.

After being on my diet for four months, patients' total cholesterol went down from 242 mg/dL to 189 mg/dL (that is a 22 percent drop) and their LDL cholesterol went from 158 mg/dL to 115 mg/dL (a 23 percent) drop. At the same time, their fasting sugar dropped from 104 mg/dL (which is an abnormally high level) to 96 mg/dL (which is normal). Finally, their weight dropped by seven pounds (3.2 kg). Those who couldn't handle the diet experienced weight, cholesterol and sugar increases!

You can see this quite dramatically illustrated in the table. There is a column called Compliant Group—Average Change Due to Diet and another column titled Noncompliant Group—Average Change. If you look at these two columns in the table you will notice something very interesting. All the numbers in the column for the compliant group have a minus sign before them because, if you kept the diet, everything went down!

Now, look at the column for the Noncompliant Group—Average Change, representing people who couldn't wean themselves off starch and saturated fat. You will see a plus sign before each number. That is because continuing to eat the way they had always eaten just made things worse.

Hmmm, losing seven pounds (3.2 kg) over four months doesn't sound like a lot for such a big change in the way you eat. You are right, it isn't a lot. But I want to draw your attention to one simple truth about the 28 people in the compliant group, who diligently and faithfully stuck to the program for four months—their baseline body mass index (BMI) was only 26.7.

Now for a brief word on BMI and you'll see the point I am trying to make and why I can state scientifically that this particular group of subjects didn't have much weight to lose to begin with.

If a Chinese physician and an American physician meet and talk about a patient's weight, as Americans are generally much fatter than Chinese, what might be considered a normal weight to the U.S. doc, may be seen as overweight to his Chinese counterpart. In other words, being fat in one country may be considered normal in another. This presents an obvious problem: if we aren't all using the same definition and may mean different things, how can we compare the weights of people from different areas of the world to one another?

Luckily, we have a scientific way of defining weight. It is called the body mass index and is a calculation that includes a person's height and weight. (You can calculate your own BMI by going online to www.nhlbisupport.com/bmi/).

A normal BMI is between 20 and 25. A person with a BMI of 25–30 is considered overweight, and if you have a BMI greater than 30, you are defined as being obese. I'll talk more about the advantages and disadvantages of BMI versus the height-to-weight ratio and body-fat composition in the next section, so don't worry if you didn't get it; we will go over the concept of BMI again.

If you look at the guys in my first study, you might be able to appreciate that the average BMI of the subjects who successfully completed my diet was only 26.7, in other words, these folks were only a little into the overweight category. They didn't have much to lose to begin with. We will soon see in the final chapter that there is a plateau phase that happens with all weight-loss diets. It often occurs when a person's weight is finally starting to trend toward the normal weight/BMI. It is those final ten pounds (4.5 kg) that just don't seem to budge despite your best efforts and behavior. So the successful group in my study was essentially starting their diet while in a plateau phase, when it is much harder to lose those last few pounds of weight. If you take everything I have just said into consideration, you will realize that even only seven of those last few pounds is still quite an accomplishment.

What I am going to tell you now is what I tell every patient that goes on my diet: Just losing weight is good, but not good enough as far as I am concerned. I want you to judge how successful this diet is based on three things happening: (1) losing weight; (2) significantly dropping your LDL cholesterol; and (3) lowering your fasting blood-glucose levels. I expect an improvement in these three areas; any less means the diet didn't work properly, and I have failed you.

Let's briefly look at my second study, published in 2015 in the same international nutrition journal, *Current Nutrition and Food Science*. This was a much larger study that included ten MDs from multiple specialties, all of whom practiced in southern Connecticut. Each MD was given ten copies of Chapter 3 of this book, which they simply handed out to their overweight, metabolic-syndrome patients. They then followed up with them 10 to 12 weeks later to see how they had gotten on.

The results of this study are very similar to the striking results of the first study, which proves that this isn't just some kind of statistical fluke but that the diet is the real deal as far as dropping weight and reversing metabolic syndrome.

Another important result from the second study is that the compliance rate in men was 74 percent compared to only 55 percent for the women. Indeed, it was this finding that convinced me that, though this lifestyle makeover works as well for women as for men, the diet is easier to keep for men, and so Man Diet was born.

At the risk of being both competitive and redundant, let's just recap what the results were of the large 2008 *New England Journal of Medicine* dietary trial that compared a low-fat diet to the Atkins diet and the Mediterranean diet. There was no change in the LDL cholesterol levels after two years on any of these three common diets. We will talk about what happened to these folks' total cholesterol levels after six years in a brief moment, but let's first look at the fasting sugar levels.

There was an improvement in fasting glucose seen in the people on the low-carb Atkins and Mediterranean groups, which is exactly what was seen in the compliant group of our own study.

Finally, we turn our attention to weight loss and note that, over the two-year study period, people on the Atkins diet lost an average of 12 pounds (5.4 kg), those on the Mediterranean diet lost ten pounds (4.5 kg) and those on the low-fat diet lost seven pounds (3.2-kg). That is obviously a greater weight loss than the seven-pound (3.2-kg) loss that we saw after four months in my first study, but not as impressive as the 14-pound (6.3-kg) weight loss over just ten weeks seen in study number two. To be fair, there are two points of view regarding how to look at the difference in weight loss seen in these studies.

On the one hand, you could argue that, as my patients were on the diet for only three to four months and they managed to lose as much weight as the people on the low-fat diet for two years, imagine how much weight they could lose after two years using my approach!

On the other hand, one could legitimately argue that this is science, not fortune-telling, and it is entirely possible that all patients re-gained all the weight, cholesterol and sugar over the subsequent two years that they had happily lost over the first three to four months.

The truth is that, as far as my first study is concerned, I was the primary care provider for all 41 patients in the study, and I can happily report that the vast majority of the successful participants subsequently modified their diets under my supervision and still managed to keep their weight, sugar and cholesterol down for a number of years afterward.

Another truism I share with all my patients is that humans need to do three things well in order to live well: eat well, sleep well and move often. You see, what you are doing on my program is a total lifestyle makeover. It's more than just a diet. I'm going to tell you exactly how to sleep, move, cope with stress and even breathe!

So get ready, my friends. By the time we are done, you will be doing all three with charm, confidence, creativity.

In case you were wondering what happened to all those people on those three famous diets, it turns out that a research group from sunny Israel published an article in the *New England Journal of Medicine* in 2012 after following the three groups for a total of six years.

The good news is that 70 percent of the people were still following their original diet (Atkins, Mediterranean or low-fat).

The less-positive news is that people did regain some of the original weight they had lost, but all in all after a total of six years, the total weight loss for those on the low-fat diet was a paltry 1.3 pounds (0.6 kg). It was a slightly better 3.7 (1.7 kg) pounds for the Atkins devotees and an almost 7-pound (3.2-kg) weight loss for the people on the Mediterranean diet.

So what happened to their cholesterol levels after six years of good behavior?

People in the low-fat group saw a 7.4 mg/dL drop in their total cholesterol. Atkins followers dropped 10.4 mg/dL in their total cholesterol levels and the Mediterranean diet people dropped 13.9 mg/dL.

For ten points, does anyone remember how much my guys' total cholesterol dropped in study 1 after four months on my eating plan? 53 mg/dL. 53 points!

Here is my point: if you look at the results of the *New England Journal* 2008 and 2012 diet studies, you'll realize that those three common weight-loss diets are just that, weight-loss diets. If losing weight isn't your only goal and you also want to drop your numbers and avoid taking medicine for your cholesterol or high sugar levels, then those diets may not be the best ones for you.

The best diet for you would, in fact, be mine.

Incidentally, of those three diets, my eating plan most closely resembles a low-calorie version of the Mediterranean diet, high in fruits, vegetables, nuts, seeds, olive oil and lean proteins. The only subtle difference between my approach and the Mediterranean diet is that initially I recommend eating less starch because, unlike the inhabitants of southern Europe, most of us are not working nine hours a day in a field or vineyard and not therefore able to burn off all that extra starch.

And make no mistake, my friends. The healthiest diet in the scientific literature is the Mediterranean one. Studies come out every month showing that it helps with diabetes, dementia and heart disease, to name but a few.

I do however always point out that the Mediterranean diet is actually a lifestyle, with a lot of activity, a good old siesta in the p.m., regular fasting for religious holidays and people commonly living in family homes with their parents, grandparents, siblings and all.

A final word on Atkins to shock and amaze, and then we'll turn our focus to the Weight Watchers study and how their results compare to mine.

A study published in the *British Medical Journal* in June 2012 looked at the health and diets of almost 44,000 Swedish women. After observing them for over fifteen years, researchers found that those on the most low-carbohydrate, high-protein Atkins-type diets had significantly increased risk of heart disease, stroke and narrowing of the arteries to the legs, a crippling disease called peripheral arterial disease, or PAD.

The researchers hypothesized that this was due to the increased saturated fat consumption that is the hallmark of an Atkins beef-burger fest, and although we have already talked about how saturated fat isn't as bad as starch and sugar, the extremely low-carbohydrate approach exemplified by Atkins and Phase 1 of the South Beach diet appears to be fraught with health dangers in the long term. Luckily, my plan is far different from the Atkins diet, so we will be dodging the heart attack and stroke if you do it my way.

I don't know about you, but these days whenever I turn on the TV there is always a former NFL superstar or other celebrity bragging about how much weight he's lost with NutriSystem, Weight Watchers or the numerous other commercially available eating plans. But is there any evidence that this stuff actually works?

Here is your answer in black and white:

In September 2011, a very interesting study was published in *The Lancet*. In Australia, Germany and the United Kingdom, 772 overweight and obese adults were divided into two groups. For one year, 377 members of the group joined the Weight Watchers program, while the other 395 people received general advice from their primary care doctor on weight loss.

Just in case any of you out there are not familiar with the famous Weight Watchers program, some key components include a reduced-calorie, balanced diet, based on healthy-living principles and a points system; increased physical activity; and weekly group meetings where you weigh yourself and see how you are progressing.

At the end of the year, 61 percent of the Weight Watchers group completed the program and filled out the 12-month assessment form, compared to 54 percent of the people who had received general advice from their GPs. The average weight loss for the Weight Watchers participants was 12 pounds (5.4 kg). The control group who received the standard medical advice on how to lose weight lost only five pounds (2.3 kg) over the same period.

At the risk of sounding like a broken record, there was yet again no statistically significant improvement in blood glucose and LDL cholesterol in the Weight Watchers group compared to the control group.

Guys, that is because a central part of Weight Watchers' strategy is to eat fewer calories, which is great if you just want to lose weight but does nothing to improve your cholesterol or sugar. Though Weight Watchers promotes a healthy diet, stresses exercise and has an organized group support system—all of which are vital components of a good weight-loss program—its diet still contains too much starch and therefore won't do all the magic you might need.

I was introduced to the merits of the whole-food, plant-based diet based on *The China Study* when I saw the award-winning documentary titled *Forks over Knives*. This 20-year study looked at dietary changes and the amount of chronic disease in 6,500 people in 65 counties in rural China.

The results were striking. People living in areas where they had adopted more Western-style eating patterns by increasing their consumption of animal proteins (dairy, eggs, poultry, meat) were more likely to die of Western diseases (heart disease, cancer, diabetes) than people living in areas where they continued eating their traditional plant-based vegan food.

I was impressed. I was so impressed that I stopped eating meat and poultry. However, before you embrace the world of veganism, there are definitely detractors to the hypothesis put forth in *The China Study*. Chief among them is Dr. Loren Cordain from Colorado State University. The father of the Paleo diet, he argues that this vegan approach is inconsistent with evolution. Remember that people were hunter-gatherers before we learned about agriculture, and that there are studies showing that consumption of lean animal protein can reduce your risk of heart disease, obesity, elevated cholesterol and high blood pressure.

You see, one of the problems in medicine is that you can pretty much find some study somewhere to support any point of view.

Studies can only take you so far. Therefore, my personal take on *The China Study* is that I don't know for sure whether lean animal protein is a good thing or a bad thing—my own diet is mostly plant-protein–based, but it still includes egg whites, low-fat dairy and a large amount of fish.

However, if meat is your thing, then as long as it is lean, you do have science supporting your dining on a juicy bison burger.

This whole argument about what our forefathers ate is a great segue into the most recent controversy surrounding the multimillion-copy best-seller *Eat Right for Your Type* by the naturopathic physician Peter J. D'Adamo.

The basic hypothesis in this book is that the ABO blood groups (every human has one of four blood types: A, B, AB or O) reveals the specific dietary habits of our ancestors, and by keeping to an eating plan that is specific to your blood type, you can improve your health and reduce your risk of developing serious illnesses like heart disease.

Let me give you two examples to help illustrate the point. According to the ABO blood group, if you have type O blood, your genetic forebearers were the good old-fashioned hunter-gatherers, replete with spears and grunts, and you should be enjoying lots of animal protein at a daily Paleo party. In contrast, if you have type A blood, then your ancestors were farmers in an agrarian society and vegetarianism should be your thing.

I have to say that the hypothesis sounds fascinating to me, and I have definitely seen people do well with some of the eating plans. However, the basic premise that our specific blood type governs exactly what diet would be best for our health has come under attack from a recently published study by researchers at the University of Toronto.

The Toronto Nutrigenomics and Health Study looked at the eating habits of 1,455 Canadians and evaluated their general health (blood pressure, cholesterol, blood glucose, weight and so on) and blood type over a one-month period. The study then tried to classify their dietary habits into one of the four blood-type eating plans to see if keeping to that diet had any impact on their health.

The researchers found that those keeping a vegetarian type A diet lost weight and improved cholesterol and blood glucose. They also found that triglycerides went down for those on the low-carb Paleo plan recommended for type O peers. Now none of this should be a surprise to you as you just read about the Paleo diet and *The China Study*.

The kicker in this research paper is that it didn't matter what the participants' blood type was. Those that kept to the vegetarian A diet got thinner on the outside and on the inside, and those that kept to the type O eating plan reduced their triglycerides, regardless of whether they had an A, O, AB or B blood type. In other words, the basic hypothesis behind the blood-type diet turned out to be incorrect.

Now, you should be aware that many supporters of the blood-type diet hypothesis have cried foul, arguing that the study was a measly one-month long and any magic takes time to reach full effect (true that!). Their other indictment was based on the way the researchers classified everyone and put them into the four different categories based on how they answered their 196-item food questionnaire.

The bottom line is that whether the hypothesis is true or false, no one can deny that people keeping to the ancient vegetarianism of our farming forefathers or to the Paleo diet of our hunter-gather predecessors may win the health lottery after all.

However, I do want to shatter one illusion that everyone has about our dear great-great-great-great-grandfather, Mr. Caveman. Our prehistoric pater was not as healthy as you might think.

In March 2013, researchers from St. Luke's Mid America Heart Institute in Kansas City published a brilliant paper in *The Lancet*. They put 137 mummies from four different areas of the globe into a CT scanner to look for signs of heart disease. Their results were shocking. Whether these prehistoric bodies came from Ancient Egypt, Peru, the Southwestern United States or Alaska, 34 percent of them already had signs of heart disease. The scientists couldn't explain this phenomenon, however they did note that all the mummies were big-time meat eaters and all shared the common element of roasting their carnivorous fare. Looks like the barbecued ribs may need to be scaled back, boys, after all; ribs may have killed off lean, mean Paleo man, so I don't rate our odds much better!

GLUTEN: A NEW FOE ON THE HORIZON

I'm sure that unless you have been living under a rock, you have heard of gluten and how everything hip and healthy is now gluten-free. But what is that all about?

Gluten is the protein found in wheat, and since wheat is found everywhere, until recently so was gluten. Now while some people are actually allergic to gluten, suffering from celiac disease, many more just can't tolerate this vegetable protein and complain of bloating and generally feeling unwell after they eat it. As feeling faint, full and flatulent is rarely fun, lots of people now opt for gluten-free fare and some notice other health benefits like weight loss to boot. Since gluten is found in wheat and wheat is a starch, my eating plan is therefore very low in gluten with an easy modification to make it entirely gluten-free. So if gluten-free is the mantra of the new you, my eating plan will help you get there.

THE ECO-ATKINS DIET

We are almost at the end of the chapter, but before I sign off, I want to tell you a little about a diet that underwent good scientific testing and showed a 20-percent drop in total cholesterol and a 21-percent drop in LDL cholesterol over four weeks. It is called the Eco-Atkins diet, and I can tell you two things about it: it works and it is really hard!

We return north of the border to Canada, to the lively city of Toronto to be more precise, where Dr. David Jenkins and colleagues recruited 47 overweight men and women with high cholesterol and hopes of better health. The participants were divided into two groups, one got a regular diet, and the other group was placed on the Eco-Atkins program. Both groups were provided only 60 percent of their daily caloric needs.

For four weeks they couldn't eat the following food: eggs, dairy, fish and poultry in addition to the usual suspects, bread, baked goods, potatoes and rice. Instead of lean animal protein, which is what you get in my diet, they all got by on protein from nuts, soy and seitan, a protein found in wheat.

The results were impressive. In addition to the significant drops in total and LDL cholesterol, there was also a nine-pound (4.1-kg) weight loss and a significant reduction in fasting sugar level. No surprise to learn that the people on the regular diet also lost nine pounds (4.1 kg) over four weeks, but their reduction in cholesterol and sugar levels were significantly less than those seen on the Eco-Atkins diet. These results are very similar to the drop in cholesterol, fasting sugar and weight that we saw in our own study but, I think you will all agree, with a much harder and more restrictive diet than ours.

Congratulations, you've done, it, you've reached the end of the most scientific section of the book. The next chapter will review the blood tests I order to get the real picture of the state of your health, and that will lead us on to a brief review of all the hormones that affect your weight, and how having the right levels can make for clear sailing into a sea of slimness and health.

2

BLOOD TESTS AND HORMONES
GETTING ALL THE FACTS

Are you a weekender woodworker? Are you the guy who spends his Saturday mornings in the garage showered in sawdust, sandpapering shelves? If that is you, then you are bound to know all about foundations and how critical they are to anything that needs to stand upright. This chapter will explain exactly how to gauge the foundations of your own health. I'll tell you what data you need to know in order for your lifestyle transformation to be successful.

On any given day, I see fifteen to twenty patients, most of whom are referred me by other local MDs for weight loss, cholesterol and sugar issues. As I said before, this is all I do for a living, and I promise you I do the same thing at the end of every first visit. I explain to the intrigued person seated in front of me that I need to get very specific laboratory tests before I give him or her the full plan. "I want to get a complete picture of your health, not just on the outside (are you fat or thin), but on the inside too," I frequently say.

This chapter deals with two vital parts of the foundation of your health. The first part goes over the tests I order so that I really know what is going on in the inside. The second part goes into a little more detail about the hormone levels that I measure and why if your levels are off, you haven't a chance of making a diet work.

BLOOD TESTS THAT LET YOU KNOW WHAT'S REALLY GOING ON

Let's begin by talking about some routine and some less routine blood tests that really help give you a picture of what's going on. Some of these blood tests are not commonly performed by doctors, and I will explain why these tests will give you more information and a better picture of your current overall health. I realize this may not be everybody's cup of tea, as it gets quite technical. If you are into science, then you will love this part; if you are less scientifically inclined, then this may be hard going and you might just skim through to get a general impression of the different tests I talk about.

THE NEW AND IMPROVED CHOLESTEROL TESTS: LDL PARTICLE NUMBER AND APOLIPOPROTEIN B LEVELS

Many people say to themselves, "As long as I can keep my cholesterol in the normal range, I won't have a heart attack." The truth is somewhat less reassuring.

Picture the scene. A 67-year-old gentleman is rushed to the local emergency room with crushing chest pain. He is panicked and sweaty and complaining that it feels like a 200-pound (90-kg) rock is crushing his chest. The emergency room physician quickly diagnoses a heart attack and this unfortunate soul rapidly finds himself on the table of the cardiac catheterization suite or in the hospital's telemetry unit on a host of new medications and with an abrupt awakening about the real state of his health. Here is the point of the story: if you were to take blood from this patient, you would be quite shocked to see that the chances are his cholesterol level would be normal!

This scary fact leads us to ask two questions: What is a normal cholesterol level? and Is the regular cholesterol panel missing something that would give us a much better idea of our actual risk of heart disease?

We'll start by answering the first question—what is a normal cholesterol level? Or put another way, what is the normal range? And who is part of this normal population?

Almost all mammals have a total cholesterol level of 150 mg/dL, and yet the average cholesterol level in American adults is 50 to 90 points higher—an impressive 200–240 mg/dL, a level still not defined as high in Western medicine.

You might argue that dogs are dogs and people are people, but the combined results of three large government population studies done over the last 35 years show that even the highest average cholesterol level you'll see in your own kids is about 170 mg/dL. This peak is usually when they are about 10 years old and the level drops back down afterward.

The numbers seen in children and other mammals are a far cry from the normal and average cholesterol numbers that I see in my adult patients every day. I therefore submit to you that a normal total cholesterol level in an adult should be the same as the levels seen in pets and children, approximately 150–160 mg/dL. And that is 150 mg/dL without being on any cholesterol-lowering medication or supplements (not so easy to achieve, unless you read this book and stick with its clinically proven program). You see, I believe that the population we should be comparing ourselves to isn't our sick, overweight neighbors, but our still (hopefully) healthy offspring. Our children may not yet have started to eat the way we do and therefore have not seen their cholesterol levels climb and their waistlines expand.

Now to the second question and a brief review of the new cutting-edge tests that are being ordered by cardiologists (heart doctors) in an effort to better assess your risk of suffering a heart attack.

A normal cholesterol panel includes four different measurements: the total cholesterol (TC); the low-density lipoprotein (LDL) are bad cholesterol; the high-density lipoprotein (HDL), or good cholesterol; and the triglycerides. This is a pretty good screening test for the general population but has limitations if you want to know your own personal risk of developing heart disease. There are a number of reasons for this, which we will now discuss.

Most people don't realize that when their doctor tells them their LDL cholesterol number, he or she is actually giving them only an estimate of their real number, based on a mathematical formula called the Friedewald equation. You can directly measure the amount of LDL in your blood, which will give you a more accurate reading of your true LDL level, but this is complex and expensive and so isn't routinely done unless you ask your doctor to order a direct LDL test.

There is also a well-known problem with the Friedewald equation: the higher your triglyceride level, the more inaccurate the estimate of your LDL level will be. To illustrate the point, if you are 50 or 100 pounds (20 or 45 kg) overweight, have a high blood glucose level, high blood pressure and low HDL cholesterol, you'll probably have high triglyceride levels too. We will talk further about what triglycerides are and why they are an important thing to measure in your blood, but for now just understand that, if your triglyceride levels are too high, your doctor won't be able to estimate your LDL cholesterol levels when he sends you for a blood test. That means both of you will be flying blind when it comes to knowing what your LDL level is, which is never a good thing.

Yet another problem with measuring the amount of cholesterol within the LDL particle is that the cholesterol content of these particles can vary among people and can be influenced by high insulin levels or high fasting glucose. In other words, if you are prediabetic or diabetic with high sugar and insulin levels, the amount of cholesterol in your type of LDL may be different from the amount seen in someone without your specific sugar challenges.

In fact, the consensus report from the American Diabetes Association and the American College of Cardiology Foundation, which appeared in the *Journal of the American College of Cardiology* in April 2008, stated that "measurement of LDL cholesterol may not accurately reflect the true burden of atherogenic particles." Or to put this into plain English, this test may not give us as accurate a picture of our actual risk of heart disease as we had thought or would like.

So what do we do?

Well, one answer is to stop worrying about LDL cholesterol levels and instead just calculate your ten-year risk of having a heart attack. If your risk is high (greater than 7.5 percent over ten years), you'll need to be on a statin medication regardless of what your LDL cholesterol level is.

And those, dear readers, are the latest (2013) and greatest new guidelines from the American Heart Association and the American College of Cardiology. Just so you know, I routinely calculate my patient's heart attack risk using an online risk calculator at the government website cvdrisk.nhlbi.nih.gov. However, I do this so I can be comfortable that we have plenty of time for a lifestyle makeover if the patient's risk is low, and we will likely avoid any cholesterol medications altogether. If, however, the risk is high, I let my patient know that the odds are we will need the prescription pad sooner rather than later.

Another way to go is to turn to a newer and more accurate test that measures LDL particle numbers using nuclear magnetic resonance (NMR) technology.

With this new test, instead of measuring the amount of LDL cholesterol (the old-school, routine cholesterol test that we have all had), the number of LDL particles is counted. This test is referred to as the LDL-P test—the P stands for the LDL particle number. Because NMR technology is used, the official name for the test and the one you should ask your doctor to order on your behalf is called an NMR LipoProfile.

The results are usually expressed in nanomoles per liter, and you ideally want your number to be under 1,000. If your level is between 1,000 and 2,000, your risk is borderline. Anything over 2,000 is high risk and therefore needs to be taken seriously.

But does all this business really make a difference?

Perhaps you believe that if your LDL cholesterol is low then you are in good shape, and if it is high, then you have a problem. Why waste all the extra money and time to be further risk stratified, as we call it in Western medicine? In other words, let's keep things simple, you propose. Ah, if only life could be simple.

Now for a scary study that will show you just how off you may be if you rely solely on your LDL cholesterol level. *The Multi-Ethnic Study of Atherosclerosis* (MESA) was published in April 2011. In this community-based observational study, 5,598 people who did not have heart disease at the start of the study were followed for a five-year period. Everybody had both a regular LDL cholesterol test and an NMR LipoProfile to count the number of LDL particles. At the end of the trial, the researchers found that, in the group of people who had normal LDL levels (less than 100 mg/dL) but had elevated LDL particle numbers (greater than 1,000 nmol/L), there was almost double the rate of having a cardiac event compared to those who had a normal number of LDL particles but elevated LDL levels.

Putting it into plain English, if your LDL particle number is high, you are at increased risk of having a heart issue; and if it is low, you are at less risk, regardless of what your LDL level is.

I don't order an NMR LipoProfile on all my patients because it is more expensive than ordering the standard cholesterol panel, and the way I see it, whether we use the plain LDL level or the flashy new LDL particle number, the number is going to go down on my diet, so the simple and cheap test often suffices.

There are, however, patients who have me a little more concerned that their risk might be higher than they think. Picture an overweight man in his early 50s who smokes and has a significant family history of heart disease. He may come to see me exclusively for weight loss, proudly proclaiming that, despite his genetics, bad dietary and daily habits, his cholesterol has never been a problem. I, however, may not be so sure and will order the NMR LipoProfile to get a better picture of what is really going on and to guide me as to whether he is really on the money as far as his cholesterol is concerned.

Now let's turn our attention to another new test on the block that is being used to assess one's risk of heart disease. North of the border, in picturesque Canada, the newest guidelines for measuring cholesterol levels now recommend adding an apolipoprotein B level to the standard cholesterol panel in patients with metabolic syndrome. Interestingly, the American College of Cardiology and the American Diabetes Association came to exactly the same conclusion in their 2008 consensus statement.

It is great that everybody is agreeing so much, but what is this apolipoprotein B test anyway, and how do I interpret my results?

I'd like to answer this question and at the same time teach you a little about cholesterol metabolism so that you will better understand why good cholesterol is good and bad cholesterol is bad. Let's begin by eating something, which is always a good idea, don't you think?

Lying before you is a handful of almonds, hard and teardrop shaped, waiting to be put in your mouth as a five o'clock snack. Yum! Before you eat this delicacy, here is a question.

What happens when you put a drop of oil into a cup of water? The oil immediately forms into little oil droplets.

The same thing happens to all the fat that we digest. It too forms into little globules in the blood. This is because fats are not soluble in water and, as blood is made up mostly of water, the fats we eat can't easily dissolve in our bloodstream, so instead they form into globules. These globules contain something else besides clumps of fat; they carry special proteins on their surfaces called apolipoproteins. These apolipoproteins make sure that the fat is eventually taken up by the right tissues of the body.

As this is medicine, we have an impressive-sounding name for these little globules of fat and protein that are wafting around in our blood vessels, and the name is one you are familiar with. They are called lipoproteins (as in low-density lipoprotein [LDL] and high-density lipoprotein [HDL]). There are different types of lipoprotein, which can be differentiated by the proportion of triglyceride and cholesterol they each contain.

Now let's return to our nut snack and watch what happens after it gets digested. The fat in the nuts is broken down into triglycerides by the enzymes in your gut and then combined with a special apolipoprotein molecule to make the first member of our lipoprotein family, the chylomicron.

Chylomicrons travel around the body in the bloodstream distributing all their triglycerides to the various tissues, where they can be used for cell structure and metabolism. Once their stores are depleted, the now empty chylomicrons make their way to the liver, where they are broken down.

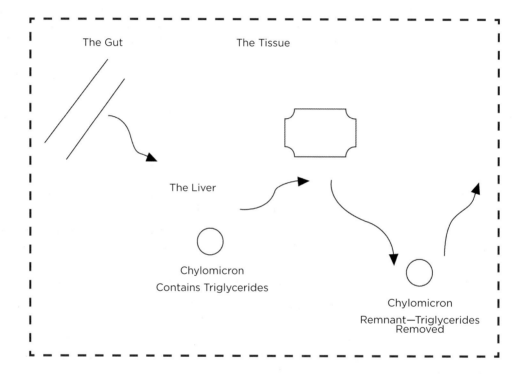

We have other lipoprotein friends that we know very well. Let's meet them and see what they actually do, and then we'll be able to understand why we call LDL bad and HDL good.

It may not surprise you to learn that 70 percent of your cholesterol is made in your body (liver), and only 30 percent comes from your diet. In fact, the entire statin class of drugs like Lipitor, Crestor, simvastatin and Pravachol work by inhibiting a special enzyme in the liver that is responsible for making cholesterol. It is no small wonder, then, that these drugs significantly drop cholesterol numbers. If 70 percent of your cholesterol is made in your body, then stopping its production will definitely lower your numbers.

Now let's look at what happens to all that cholesterol that is made by the body, and then we shall be able to understand what LDL, HDL and even VLDL particles are.

It all starts with the liver, the body's own special cholesterol factory. The liver makes cholesterol and triglycerides and neatly packages them together with some apolipoproteins (one of which is called apo B) into our second particle of the day—the VLDL particle.

VLDL particles are similar in composition to the chylomicrons that we have just heard about. VLDL and chylomicrons are both made mostly of triglycerides, but with a critical difference between them. The triglycerides found in chylomicrons come from the fat that we eat, whereas the triglycerides found in VLDL particles are made in our livers.

Very nice, you might be thinking, but who cares about VLDL and chylomicrons anyway? I care. And so should you.

In February 2011, a large Danish study called the Copenhagen City Heart Study published its findings. The researchers analyzed data from 7,500 women and 6,300 men over a two-year period. They found that women with the highest triglyceride levels had nearly a four-times greater risk of having a stroke compared to those with the lowest triglyceride levels. Since the major carriers of triglycerides in the bloodstream are the chylomicrons and VLDL particles, you can now see why knowing about VLDL and chylomicrons could prove clinically relevant.

Putting it another way, having high levels of these particles in your bloodstream can increase your risk of having a stroke by 400 percent!

Interestingly enough, current stroke-prevention guidelines only consider LDL cholesterol levels and don't yet recommend a goal for triglyceride levels. Perhaps that will change.

This shiny new VLDL particle, packed with triglycerides, cholesterol and its apolipoproteins, is released into the bloodstream and begins its journey around the body, where it supplies the various tissue with all its goodies. When the VLDL particle reaches muscle tissue, for example, it gives triglycerides to the muscles to use as fuel. If the VLDL particle arrives at some adipose tissue (fat), the VLDL will offer up its triglycerides to the fat cells, where they will be stored for future energy needs—and we get fatter!

Once the VLDL particle has given up its triglycerides and is now composed mostly of cholesterol, it will be smaller and denser, and it will acquire a new name, a name that we have all grown to recognize and fear, the one and only LDL.

So what is so bad about LDL? The answer is that nothing is ever just bad, except for maybe trans fats and Twinkies!

LDL particles have many important functions. They can be taken up by cells and their cholesterol can then be used to make cell membranes, hormones and other good things.

However, the LDL particles can also be taken up into the walls of your arteries, where they will cause your blood vessels to narrow. Narrowing of the blood vessels is what causes heart attacks, strokes and peripheral arterial disease (PAD). It is for this reason that we can call LDL cholesterol bad.

Many people, and some physicians, don't think LDL cholesterol has anything to do with heart disease and feel that the obsession by other physicians to bring down everybody's cholesterol levels with a small white pill is due to conspiracy and collusion between the drug companies and doctors. Many argue that, in fact, heart disease is caused by inflammation, not elevated cholesterol, and we are all missing the mark on the target we are trying to treat.

I like to play nicely with everyone in the sandbox, but if we are going to work together, then you should be aware of my position on this important issue. I have no doubt that inflammation plays a critical role in many diseases, including heart disease. We will talk about the tests I run for inflammation in a few pages. I also feel that there is enough evidence in the medical literature to implicate LDL cholesterol as a factor in heart disease. I just don't believe for a millisecond that we all need a pill to get down to 150. I think the vast majority of people don't need any cholesterol medications at all, ever (I haven't prescribed a statin in almost five years). They need to learn to eat, move, sleep, love and laugh. They need a real lifestyle makeover, and that is just what you are getting. Lucky you!

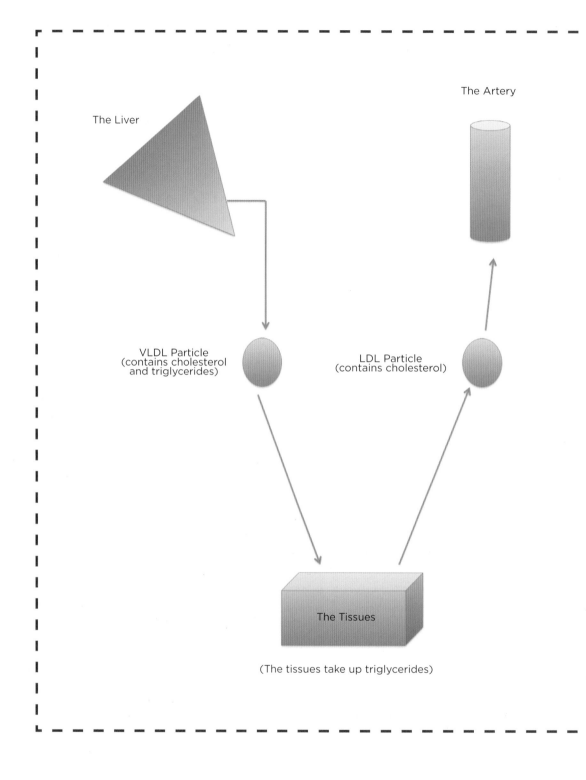

The Artery

The Liver

VLDL Particle
(contains cholesterol
and triglycerides)

LDL Particle
(contains cholesterol)

The Tissues

(The tissues take up triglycerides)

We are almost done, but I still haven't described what the apo B test actually is and why it is really helpful.

As I said before, every type of lipoprotein has its own special apolipoprotein "best friend" that it hangs around with. The LDL cholesterol particle is no exception, and its special protein buddy is called apolipoprotein B.

Now the next bit is very important so please read it carefully!

You know the old saying that you can only have one best friend? Well this rings particularly true in the case of LDL and apo B. Each and every LDL particle has a single apolipoprotein B attached to it. Therefore, if we measure the apo B level, it is essentially the same as measuring the number of LDL particles in the bloodstream.

We learned before that knowing the number of LDL particles is more useful for assessing risk of heart disease than just measuring the concentration of LDL in the blood. Now you can clearly see why the apo B level is useful to know. It is no small wonder that all those professional bodies like the American College of Cardiology and American Diabetes Association now recommend measuring it.

Now what is so good about HDL? The answer is simple: HDL cholesterol particles that are also made in the liver do exactly the opposite that LDL particles do. They pick up the cholesterol that is going to the arteries and other tissues, and take it straight back to the liver. To better understand this, let me use the garbage analogy one of my patients once told me. If the LDL particles are like garbage, then the HDL particles are like garbage collectors. If you want your streets to be clean, you need to employ enough garbage collectors (HDL) to clear away the trash (LDL). In fact, there are multiple clinical studies showing that in both diabetic and nondiabetic people, high levels of HDL cholesterol (greater than 60 mg/dL) are associated with significantly less risk of having heart disease.

IT IS ALL ABOUT THE SUGAR: GLYCATED HEMOGLOBIN AND FASTING INSULIN LEVELS

I am not joking. It really is all about the sugar. There is an epidemic of people in the United States with blood glucose issues. This can run the gamut from mildly elevated fasting blood glucose in a marginally overweight person to a brutal type 2 diabetic who has burned out his or her pancreas completely and only survives by injecting insulin daily.

I would like to introduce you to the most current research on glycated hemoglobin and fasting insulin levels, and explore why these tests are needed in addition to the standard fasting sugar test that is ordered by most doctors. If you already have diabetes, you will be quite familiar with the glycated hemoglobin test. This is a blood test that gives you an idea of how high your blood glucose levels have been for the last three months. It is now the standard of care for all diabetic patients to have their glycated hemoglobin, or HbA1c, tested every three months. In fact, this is one of the main tests your doctor relies on to decide how well controlled your diabetes is. All the trials on the newest diabetes drugs always test HbA1c levels, and pharmaceutical manufacturers predictably try to show a significant drop in HbA1c levels using their new and improved products.

Without getting too technical, the test measures the percentage of hemoglobin in your blood that has become glycated by being exposed over a long period of time to the sugar in your blood. Putting it into plainer English, here is how the test works: Hemoglobin is made up of proteins and iron. When it is exposed to sugar over a long period of time, it becomes chemically altered. This chemically altered hemoglobin is called glycated hemoglobin. Now, perhaps you can begin to see how this test works. The higher the sugar level has been in your blood over the previous three months, the more chemically altered, glycated hemoglobin will be found when this blood test is done.

I test HbA1c levels on many of my patients and often find that they are higher than expected. Once I have explained to them what a HbA1c test actually is, everyone usually wants to know what is the normal range for an HbA1c level in the same way they ask for the normal range for cholesterol levels.

Unfortunately, the answer is a little more complex as the goalposts for the normal range move depending upon whom you ask.

Let's look at some facts on HbA1c levels and then decide for ourselves.

In 2009, the International Expert Committee, which represents several major diabetes groups, recommended using an HbA1c test as a new and additional way to diagnose diabetes. Previously, we had all been diagnosing the disease based solely on blood glucose levels. The new critical level to be diagnosed as diabetic was decided to be an HbA1c of greater than 6.5 percent. (Incidentally, in 2013 this recommendation was also adopted by two more large medical societies: the European Society of Cardiology and the European Association for the Study of Diabetes.) If an HbA1c level greater than 6.5 percent is diabetic, then what is the prediabetic range?

In January 2011, Ronald Ackerman and colleagues reported the results of an important study in the *American Journal of Preventive Medicine* that helps answer that very question. They studied data from the National Health and Nutrition Examination Survey (NHANES) 2003–2006 population study. The researchers looked at people who had been diagnosed as prediabetic using the older criteria (based on blood glucose levels) and saw what percentage of those people actually went on to develop diabetes over the following seven years. The answer was that 34 percent of them did.

Now for the clever part. They then relooked at those same people, but this time instead of using blood glucose levels to diagnose prediabetes, they used HbA1c level. The results were very interesting. Using an HbA1c level of greater than 5.7 percent as the new criterion for diagnosing prediabetes, the probability of developing full-blown diabetes over the next seven years was 41 percent.

Putting it simply, the HbA1c test picked up more people (41 percent) at risk of diabetes than the older blood glucose test (34 percent) did. And that's why I test HbA1c levels on all people with only slightly high fasting glucose levels (greater than 100 mg/dL).

So where are we now?

We can conclude, based on the above study, that any HbA1c greater than 5.7 percent is abnormal and puts you at an increased risk of diabetes. In fact, an HbA1c level of greater than 5.7 percent is now considered abnormal by most physicians, and most laboratories would report this result as abnormally high. Therefore, most physicians would say that any HbA1c less than 5.7 percent is normal and nothing to worry about.

To summarize, here are the HbA1c ranges for diabetes, prediabetes and normal according to Western medicine; greater than 6.5 percent = diabetes, 5.7–6.4 percent = prediabetes, and less than 5.7 percent is normal.

But hold the press. There is a glitch in the works regarding what is really a normal HbA1c level.

Two VA medical centers analyzed the charts of more than 12,000 former servicemen and -women who were not diabetic at the start of the study. All of these veterans had had their HbA1c levels tested and so the researchers then looked at what happened to these 12,000 people over a subsequent four years. They found that if these people had an HbA1c greater than 5.0 percent, they had an almost twofold-increased risk of developing diabetes over the next four years, compared to those who were lucky enough to have an HbA1c level of less than 5.0 percent. If their HbA1c level was between 5.5 and 5.9 percent, the risk was five times greater, and if they started with an HbA1c of between 6.0 and 6.4 percent, the risk was a whopping 16 times greater than if they had an HbA1c level of less than 5.0 percent at the start of the study. In other words, according to the VA study, any HbA1c level greater than 5.0 percent puts you at increased risk of diabetes! That is quite a different story from the 5.7 percent cutoff that most physicians still regard as a normal level for this blood test.

So to ask the question again, what is a "normal" HbA1c level? I think the answer is that it should be optimally less than 5.0 percent. Anything bordering 5.7, like 5.5 or 5.6 percent, may already be the beginning of a sugar problem.

Now that you know all about HbA1c levels and how you can easily tell whether you have normal blood glucose or are already be prediabetic, I want to comment on a practice I regularly see and always condemn.

Patients quite often present me with their labs and tell me that their physician has told them not to worry about them. While it is true that many abnormal readings on lab tests are not significant and will be completely normal the next time you are tested, an elevated HbA1c is not something to ignore or downplay. Here is why:

In 2013, endocrinologists from all over the United States congregated in sun-bathed Phoenix, Arizona, at the annual meeting of the American Association of Clinical Endocrinologists. At this gathering, researchers from Wayne State University in Detroit presented a paper on the risk of having heart disease if you had prediabetes. They found that 36 percent of people with prediabetes already had heart disease when they underwent coronary catheterization (putting a tube in the groin and then squirting dye into the arteries of the heart to see if they are blocked) compared to an only slightly higher 42 percent of the truly diabetic patients.

The bottom line is that if you are prediabetic, you have a problem, and as the study above demonstrated, you may already have heart disease, so don't shrug this one off!

Having read Chapter 1, you are now aware of how significant the storage hormone insulin is to your weight, sugar and cholesterol woes. It stands to reason that measuring an insulin level in the morning before you have eaten anything would give you some useful information. Remember that if you have insulin resistance, the cells in your body will only be sluggishly responding to your insulin, and your pancreas will be forced to make abnormally high amounts of it. A high fasting insulin level would, therefore, be a useful marker for insulin resistance.

We now circle back once more to our favorite question of this section, the one we have asked about every laboratory test we have talked about so far: What is the normal range for the test we have ordered? So what is a normal fasting insulin level? And the answer is—drum roll, please . . .

According to the NHANES III data, the average insulin level in the population is between 9 and 11 microunits/ml. Based on that fact, I aim for all my patients' fasting insulin levels to be ideally under 10, once they have reached their ideal body weight using my diet. Many of my patients will start off with levels in the 20 to 30 range, and I even had one poor police officer who rolled in with a fasting insulin level of over 120! I am delighted to say he is doing much better now, his insulin dropped from 120 to 37 with a 30-pound (13.6-kg) weight loss after only two to three months on the program. He now has a much longer and health-filled life to look forward to. He also sent me half the local police force because of his new look, so it was really a win-win all around.

THE LATEST ON CARDIAC CRP AND HOMOCYSTEINE LEVELS

It is quite fascinating how our bodies react to different stresses. Too much heat from the sun, irritating rubbing from a tight-fitting shoe or even a drop of hot oil on our skin will all result in the same thing: inflammation. The inflamed area of the body will become red, hot, swollen and painful—an experience we know all too well from the many times we have injured ourselves in the past.

We now know that heart disease is also caused by inflammation, but this time it is inflammation in the lining of the blood vessels. We can get an idea of the amount of inflammation that exists inside those inflamed blood vessels using a special blood test called a cardiac CRP. But before you all go out and request this expensive test from your primary-care physician, it is worth noting that this test is controversial. Canadian cardiologists recommend using this test to help them better evaluate the risk of heart disease in their patients. American cardiologists, however, are still on the fence about how useful this test is to help gauge the risks of having heart disease. Some of the problems with cardiac CRP are that the levels vary depending upon your race and sex, or if you have inflammation anywhere in your body for any other reason (such as having inflamed gums or a nasty cold), the results can be abnormally high. Generally speaking, we interpret the results of this test as follows: Less than 1 mg/L is defined as low risk of heart disease. With cardiac CRP levels between 1 and 3 mg/L, the risk is a little higher; and levels greater than 3 mg/L put you at the highest risk. I use this test with patients who appear to have normal cholesterol levels but with whom I suspect there is more going on. I will often use a high dose of fish oil (EPA/DHA greater than 1,200–1,500 mg per day) in addition to my diet, as a way to quickly reduce the inflammation in those hot and angry blood vessels.

Homocysteine is an amino acid produced by the body through the conversion of another amino acid called methionine that is found in the meat products we eat. Since the 1990s, physicians have noted that high homocysteine levels in the blood tend to be associated with an increased risk of developing heart disease and stroke. We still aren't sure how homocysteine affects blood vessels, and the unfortunate news from multiple studies is that lowering your homocysteine levels doesn't appear to reduce your subsequent risk of having heart problems. Nevertheless, the latest research suggests that this test can help better assess your risk of heart disease, as we shall hear about below.

The paper on homocysteine appeared in the August 2011 edition of the *Journal of the American College of Cardiology*. The researchers in this paper analyzed data from two population studies with which we are already very familiar. Please welcome again to the stage our old favorites, the NHANES III study and the MESA study (which I told you about earlier in this chapter when we discussed the advantages of the LDL particle number over the standard LDL test).

These researchers, again from Wayne State University in Detroit, started their research by defining an elevated homocysteine level as one greater than 15 micromoles/L. They then assessed all the people at the start of both the NHANES III study and the MESA study for their risk of developing heart disease using just the traditional risks factors such as age, smoking, diabetes, hypertension, family history and so on.

Next they observed what happened to those people over the subsequent six years in the MESA study and over fifteen years for the NHANES III participants. Finally, they reassessed everybody's numbers from the start of the study, but this time they factored in their baseline homocysteine levels and watched to see how adding this extra piece of information would change the people's risk of developing heart trouble over those same ensuing years. Here is what they found:

Those who had a high homocysteine level of greater than 15 millimoles/L at the start of the study, even after adjusting and accounting for the traditional risks factors, had a 2.6 higher risk of dying from heart disease than if they had a normal (less than 15 millimoles/L) homocysteine level.

The authors concluded their paper by stating that their study "provides a sound rationale for adding homocysteine in cardiovascular risk assessment." I couldn't agree more, could you?

BMI, WAIST-TO-HEIGHT RATIO AND BODY FAT ANALYSIS—NO BLOOD REQUIRED

Remember how in Chapter 1 I described how physicians from all parts of the world use the same measurement to categorize their patients as underweight, normal weight, overweight or obese? This measurement is a simple formula called the **body mass index** (BMI), which is your weight in kilograms divided by your height in meters, squared. With it you can work out whether your weight is healthy or not, and what your goal weight should be. You have probably even been shown those colored BMI tables that people use to compare you to others of similar height—something that is not always very productive, as you will read about below.

I freely admit that I use BMI all the time as a rough gauge for how far we have to go and how many pounds we have to shed together, but I do often find myself explaining the limitations of this measurement so that my patients don't get obsessed with some unattainable number that is both unrealistic and unpleasant to try to reach.

The most striking problem with the BMI is that it assumes that everybody of the same height has the same build. That is clearly preposterous. Just think back to your college football team and the difference in build between the wide receivers and the offensive linemen, who may all have been exactly the same height.

There are many ways to be 6 feet 2 inches (1 m 88 cm) tall. You can look like a bean pole or be built like a Calvin Klein model, but based on BMI, everyone who is 6 feet 2 inches (1 m 88 cm) needs to be in a rather narrow weight range to be considered normal, regardless of their build. That is why body builders are often overweight or obese on BMI charts, the formula doesn't account for build or muscle mass.

This leads us to a study published in *PLOS ONE* in 2012 that compared BMI to direct measurement of body fat (aka body fat analysis) in 1,400 adults seen at a NYC wellness center. The researchers found that 25 percent of men who were obese according to their BMI were not actually obese when you measured their percentage of body fat (a normal body fat composition in men is less than 24 percent). There are two points to consider:

- Before we all throw away the BMI charts and assume that we all actually look like Adonis, the same study showed that 39 percent of people who had normal BMI were in fact obese when they measured their body fat (a medical condition called normal BMI obesity) or thin, but were all fat and no muscle. The study used a flashy dual emission X-ray absorptiometry machine, a toy that is hard to come by for most guys. Luckily, there are some low-tech versions of that machine that can give you an estimate of your body fat composition. They use the difference in how fat vs. muscle conducts electricity and can safely tell you what you are made of, all for a low price at your local big-box store.
- The other measurement I use is the waist-to-height ratio (WHtR), which helps me guide weight-loss goals so that my patient slims down in the right places (belly and love handles, not pecs and quads). The basic idea is that your waist in inches should be less than or equal to half your height in inches. For example, I am a short 5 feet 6 inches (1 m 70 cm). I hate it but what can I do? Unless I want to be stretched out a little on a medieval rack, I'm stuck being a taller and much less colorful member of the Oompa Loompa tribe. I am therefore a towering and formidable 66 inches (168 cm), so my waist size, pants size and belt size should all be less than or equal to 33 inches (84 cm). And the science, is with me . . .

In May 2013, scientists presented a paper to an international obesity conference in Liverpool, England. They analyzed data from two large British health surveys and looked at the risk of dying over time using the BMI vs. the WHtR. Their results are striking: those who have a BMI of 40 (morbid obesity) have a life expectancy that is 10.5 years shorter than someone of the same age with a normal BMI.

The life expectancy of a morbidly obese person as defined by the WHtR is 16.7 years shorter than that of a person with a normal WHtR. The researchers concluded that the WHtR is a more accurate indicator of mortality risk.

The bottom line is that you want to follow both your BMI and WHtR and watch them drop together because the evidence suggests you'll live a lot longer!

Before I end this first part, I do want to state that you do not need to have every single blood test I have talked about before you begin my diet. What I hope I have given you is an overview of some of the latest tests that are available to help both you and your doctor work out what is really going on inside as well as outside.

THOSE DAMNED HORMONES AGAIN!

Hormones, hormones, hormones. They control so many fundamental processes in our bodies, like growth, fertility, libido (also known as sex drive, boys), metabolism and, of course, weight. They are chemicals that are made in specialized glands and are vitally important to your survival. In this section, we'll talk about a number of hormones and their relationship to metabolism and weight control. You'll also see how you have no chance of losing an ounce if their numbers are off!

TESTOSTERONE

What makes you a man? It is a good question. Most people would answer that it is because you have a penis and testicles dangling between your legs. What is interesting to note is that all fetuses (babies very early in their development) are preprogrammed to automatically become female (who is the dominant sex now, my friends?)

So how did 50 percent of us end up as boys? The answer is simple. Some fetuses start producing a hormone called testosterone, and this fantastic chemical helps them develop testes, a prostate and a penis. This very same testosterone is the reason men have a larger muscle mass than women and more body hair. In other words, the hormone testosterone, made in our testes, wafts throughout our body making us big, buff, hairy and horny!

Testosterone is a vital part of your mojo, and when your levels are low, it isn't just your sex drive that is down, it also makes you fat on the inside and the outside!

A study in Finland in 2004 that went on for 11 years and included over 700 middle-aged men found that men with the lowest levels of testosterone had at least twice the risk of developing diabetes or metabolic syndrome compared to the other men.

And trust me, my brothers. Our Finnish friends with low testosterone didn't look so hot either. But I have an even better visual for you. When was the last time you went to a beach? Do you remember seeing any heavyset men with man boobs? I am sure you did. And I bet you thought to yourself, "what the hell is all that about?"

Want to know why these poor guys have breast tissue that some women would be envious of? It turns out that if you are an obese male, much of that lovely testosterone you make is turned into the female hormone estrogen by your fat cells! In other words, fat men turn into fat women. How is that for a visual?

It gets worse.

In May 2013 at the European Congress of Endocrinology, researchers from Ghent University in Belgium reported the results of a small study of 20 healthy young men who were given medicine to put them into male menopause and increase their estrogen levels. What they found was that the changes in testosterone and estrogen that are typically seen in obesity (low testosterone and high estrogen—all woman and no man) caused significant abnormalities in their heart function, and this was after only one week. Now imagine what 30 years of low testosterone and high estrogen will do to your body! Not pretty.

So, if low testosterone is so bad for you, then the obvious next questions are how can I raise my testosterone levels, and will raising my testosterone levels help with metabolic syndrome and my low sex drive?

Yes, yes and yes are the short answers! Let's look at the details.

Eighty-one diabetic men with low testosterone were randomly put into two groups for six months and given either testosterone injections or a placebo. At the end of the six months they found that the guys who had received the testosterone had a "dramatic" 25-percent increase in insulin sensitivity (all their cells became more responsive to their body's own insulin—we'll talk about this is a few pages). Those in the placebo group had no change.

Over 30 percent of all diabetic men have low testosterone, therefore getting a little testosterone replacement appears to be good not only for their sex life but also for their sugar!

But now for some cautions.

Testosterone levels naturally drop in men as they age. For example, a 75-year-old man has a total testosterone level about two-thirds less than he did when he was 20 or 30. Let us also not forget that the diabetic patients in these studies all have low testosterone, based on a level of less than 300 mg/dL. So if your testosterone level is clearly in a normal range, then taking extra testosterone isn't appropriate. Why take more of what you already have enough of?

Most MDs who treat men with low testosterone would agree that, if your levels are low and you have symptoms, you should be on replacement therapy.

A problem arises with men who have normal testosterone levels but vague symptoms of dwindling vitality, who want a fountain of youth injected into their posterior every two weeks. Using testosterone replacement in these gentlemen is controversial.

There are also clear risks associated with using testosterone therapy. Problems with your liver and breast swelling or tenderness start off the list. Testosterone increases the amount of red blood cells in your bloodstream, causing the blood to become more viscous and making it easier for blood clots to form.

Then there is the whole question about prostate cancer, whose growth can be enhanced by all that extra testosterone. To be fair, there is evidence on both sides of the argument regarding whether testosterone replacement increases the risk of prostate cancer.

And now there are the latest studies published in January 2014 by researchers at the National Cancer Institute that analyzed the data on over 55,000 men and found that in men older than 65, testosterone replacement doubled their risk of having a heart attack within the first six months of taking the medication. The same was also seen in younger men who had a known history of heart disease.

However you look at it, testosterone replacement in men has risks, just as hormone replacement therapy does in women. So use caution with this purported panacea of youth—it can have a bite.

THE THYROID

People come to my office every day with thyroid problems—most of them are women, but some are men. They all recite that well-known medical fact that it is much harder to lose weight and lower sugar and cholesterol if your thyroid gland isn't working properly. The tricky part is how you define a normal-functioning thyroid. So let's talk about the concept of a low-functioning thyroid, or subclinical hypothyroidism, an autoimmune condition that affects roughly 13 million Americans and often goes untreated by the Western medical establishment.

The thyroid is a small, bow-tie-shaped, 15 gram gland found in the neck that is responsible for the rate of metabolism, something that clearly is critical to weight loss. It produces two hormones: Thyroxine (T4), which lasts in the body for seven to ten days, and triiodothyronine (T3), which is much more active and lasts only hours in the circulatory system before being metabolized. T4 is converted in the tissues to the much more metabolically active T3.

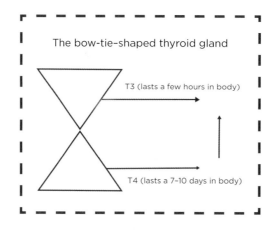

The bow-tie-shaped thyroid gland

T3 (lasts a few hours in body)

T4 (lasts a 7-10 days in body)

Simple so far, I hope!

You may be wondering how the thyroid gland decides how much of its thyroid hormones to release into the bloodstream. The answer is that it doesn't decide!

Everybody in life has a boss. I have many; at top of the list would be my wife, obviously. The thyroid gland is no exception. It too has a "boss" who tells it when to make more of its hormones and when to make less of them. The boss of the thyroid is a gland called the pituitary, which sits at the very center of the brain and is the overall boss of all the body's various hormones.

The pituitary gland controls the thyroid by producing a hormone called thyroid stimulating hormone (TSH), which does exactly what its name implies and stimulates the thyroid to make and release the two thyroid hormones.

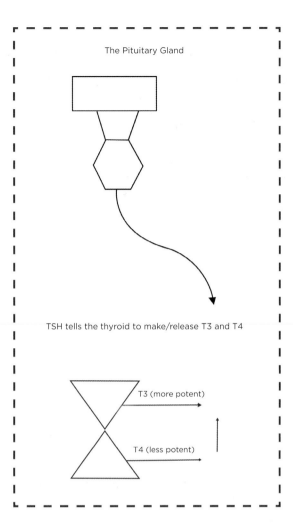

The Pituitary Gland

TSH tells the thyroid to make/release T3 and T4

T3 (more potent)

T4 (less potent)

Once the two thyroid hormones are released into the blood, the pituitary senses an increase in the hormone levels and makes less TSH. This is called a negative feedback loop and is the way that the pituitary gland controls every hormone level in our body. If we had no feedback loop, the pituitary gland would continue to stimulate the thyroid to make more and more hormone, regardless of the amount of hormone already in the blood, and the levels would quickly turn toxic. And what would that look like? That would look like hyperthyroidism and you would be anxious, sweaty, tired, nervous and at risk of developing abnormal heart rhythms—not fun at all.

Below is a picture of the negative feedback loop that shows how the amount of TSH the pituitary makes will depend upon how much T3 and T4 the thyroid is making.

To go back to the boss analogy, if you do your work and your boss sees the results, he leaves you alone. Similarly, if the thyroid produces sufficient amounts of T3 and T4, the pituitary will see it in the blood and reduce the amount of TSH that it releases.

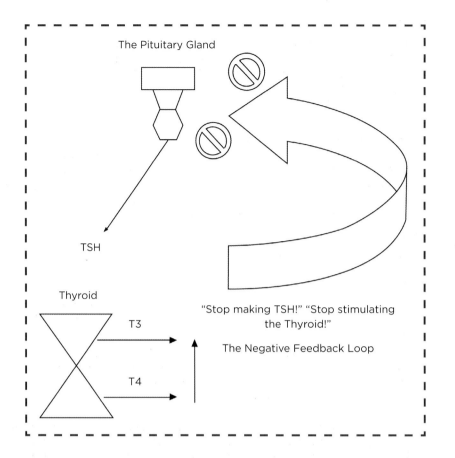

The Pituitary Gland

TSH

Thyroid

T3

T4

"Stop making TSH!" "Stop stimulating the Thyroid!"

The Negative Feedback Loop

Now let's look at what happens to this neat little control system when the thyroid doesn't function properly.

If your thyroid is sick, it will struggle to produce T4 and T3, and the levels of these thyroid hormones in the blood will dip. The pituitary gland, sensing this dip, will increase its production of TSH to try to return the thyroid hormone levels to normal. There is a name for when your thyroid gland is slow. It is called hypothyroidism.

According to the NHANES III study, 4.6 percent of the population has hypothyroidism, defined as a TSH level greater than 4.5 mIU/L in the blood. That would translate to roughly 14 million Americans in the current population. That's a lot of people who won't be able to lose weight or drop their cholesterol because their thyroid is off and their metabolism is too slow. The NHANES study found that hypothyroidism is much more common in women, increases with age and is seen most often in Caucasians and Mexican Americans.

The study also found that in the vast majority of people who have hypothyroidism, even though they have elevated TSH levels, the levels of their thyroid hormones are still normal. This condition is now called subclinical hypothyroidism, according to the American Thyroid Association. If you recall, subclinical hypothyroidism occurs when the TSH level is high but the thyroid hormone levels in the blood are still within the normal range.

How can that happen?

The answer is simple. Let's first remember that the earliest and most sensitive indicator of an underactive thyroid is an elevated TSH level. In subclinical hypothyroidism, the pituitary needs to stimulate the struggling little thyroid gland more than usual in order to maintain a normal level of circulating thyroid hormones. The TSH level therefore rises, while the T3 and T4 levels are still managing to stay in the normal range. Unfortunately, the thyroid will eventually get too sick, and the levels of T3 and T4 in the blood will drop, resulting in clinical hypothyroidism.

Most people don't care too much about this elegant dance of hormone levels in the blood. What people really want to know is whether they will develop any problems if they have subclinical hypothyroidism. In fact, many patients with subclinical hypothyroidism will start to experience the symptoms associated with an underactive thyroid, such as weight gain, fatigue, cold intolerance, hair loss and problems with memory. They might also see a rise in their bad cholesterol and a worsening of their diabetes, if they suffer from that disease. And even more concerning, people with subclinical hypothyroidism have an increased risk of heart disease.

I'm as serious as a heart attack.

So clearly, subclinical hypothyroidism doesn't sound like much fun.

Do you want to know what causes it?

Every medical textbook states that the most common cause of hypothyroidism is an autoimmune condition called Hashimoto's thyroiditis, where the body's own immune system attacks the thyroid gland, slowly causing it to stop functioning normally.

Hashimoto's disease is quite simple to diagnose because there is an autoantibody called antithyroperoxidase antibody (anti-TPO Ab) that is seen in 70–90 percent of patients with the disease, and you can therefore see if you have this special antibody in your blood by undergoing a simple blood test.

So if you have the test and it comes out positive, what does that mean?

It means, my friends, that you have a significantly increased risk of eventually developing hypothyroidism. In fact, other clinical studies put the risk of developing full-blown hypothyroidism at 5 percent per year if you have a positive anti-TPO Ab blood test together with an elevated TSH of greater than 4.5 mIU/L.

In my own practice, all patients who are seen for weight loss are sent for a full thyroid panel as well as the anti-TPO Ab test (if they have a family history of thyroid issues). Anyone who has an elevated TSH, problems losing weight and a positive anti-TPO Ab test is treated for subclinical hypothyroidism.

The obvious next question is how?

The standard treatment of subclinical hypothyroidism is supplementing the thyroid hormones your body makes with extra synthetic or natural thyroid hormones. This little bit extra thyroid hormone boosts the levels in the blood, and the pituitary, sensing that the blood levels have returned to normal, stops overproducing TSH, and the TSH levels return to the normal range. It is for this reason that most Western physicians only need to rely on the TSH level to decide how much thyroid hormone replacement to give someone.

Now are you all wondering from where we obtain these thyroid replacement medications? There are two main sources—a natural one and a synthetic one. Mother Nature is kind. In order to obviate the necessity for us to all butcher each other in a foolhardy attempt to get the extra thyroid hormones that we require, she has provided us with another natural source of thyroid hormones—the pig. If you prefer the vegetarian option on the menu, there are always synthetic thyroid hormones that are made in the chemistry laboratory.

Many patients prefer the natural thyroid replacement as it contains both T4 and T3 and is authentic thyroxine and triiodothyronine, as opposed to the chemical versions found in the synthetic preparations. Opponents of the natural hormone replacement argue that the pig thyroid tissue also contains proteins that are foreign to our bodies and could cause some kind of immune reaction when taken. They also charge that it is hard to ensure that the dosage will be exactly the same between batches.

Clinically, I don't feel that there is much advantage to one type of preparation over the other, and I really go according to the patient's individual preference, sometimes compounding either type of medicine for a more individualized dose.

By the way, just in case the whole heart attack thing passed you by, I was serious. There is an increased risk of developing heart disease if you have subclinical hypothyroidism.

The good news is that a huge seven-year study of over 5,500 Brits with subclinical hypothyroidism showed that, if you treat the condition with thyroid medicine, you are much less likely to actually have some kind of heart event, especially if you are younger than 70 years old. Sounds like we should all get going with those pills, people!

Just to finish off, in the world of alternative medicine, in addition to using thyroid hormone replacement, two minerals are routinely recommended to help treat hypothyroidism. Let's briefly look at the evidence for both these mineral supplements: iodine and selenium.

Iodine is a vital mineral found in rocks and seawater. Its name comes from the Greek word for *purple*, which is the color of the gas it turns into when heated. Iodine is found in high concentrations in kelp, a type of seaweed that is taken by many people with thyroid problems. This substance is the building block of the two thyroid hormones, and in inland areas of the world where there is little seafood eaten, iodine deficiency and hypothyroidism are commonplace. In fact, lack of iodine during pregnancy causes the baby to develop hypothyroidism while still in the womb, something that leads to severe mental retardation, or cretinism, when the baby is born. Iodine is therefore essential for normal thyroid function. However, as is the case with all micronutrients, there is an optimal level, and problems can develop if you take too much.

In order for the thyroid gland to make the required daily amount of T4 and T3, it needs only 70 micrograms of iodine. Interestingly, the recommended daily amount as per the Institute of Medicine is around 150 micrograms, which is double what the thyroid actually needs, because the iodine is also used in many other tissues in the body.

Do average Americans get enough iodine in their diet, you may be thinking? Well, according to the United States National Research Council, the answer is yes! Its research in 2000 showed that the average daily intake of iodine from food in the USA was 240–300 micrograms daily for men and 190–210 micrograms for women. Clearly, then, the average American does not need to add any extra iodine by taking kelp supplements, though many in the alternative world believe that the 150 microgram daily requirement set by the government is too low and recommend supplementing with 500 or even 1,000 micrograms daily.

Selenium is another trace mineral that is necessary for optimal health. It is incorporated into proteins to make selenoproteins, which are vital for the production of thyroid hormones, as well as for proper immune function and the making of antioxidants for the body. Plant foods are the major dietary sources of selenium, especially Brazil nuts, but selenium is also found in tuna, cod and turkey, along with some other meats and seafood. The level of selenium in food depends upon the amount of selenium in the soil, and this can vary considerably from the record high levels in Nebraska to the minimal levels in some areas of China and Russia.

According to the Institute of Medicine, the recommended daily allowance for selenium is 50 micrograms, and the NHANES III survey indicated that most Americans achieve that level in their diets. However, integrative physicians again question whether the 50 microgram level is too low. They cite a large amount of emerging data that shows a reduction in certain kinds of cancer, such as bladder and colon, with doses in the 100–200 microgram range. Supplementation above 400 micrograms is not recommended, and there is at least some evidence from a 2008 analysis of the original NHANES III data suggesting that a high blood selenium level may be associated with an increased death rate, again illustrating the point that too much of anything is never a good thing.

You may note that I specifically asked about eating foods that are naturally high in selenium, rather than taking supplements. Let's just talk about dietary supplements for a second and see why food is always preferable to pills. Hippocrates stated, "Let thy food be thy medicine," a teaching I subscribe to whenever possible. To illustrate the wisdom of this maxim I will refer to a clinical trial that appeared in the February 2008 issue of the *American Journal of Clinical Nutrition*. In this study, 59 New Zealand adults were divided into three groups. One group was given 100 mcg of selenium as a pill, one got two Brazil nuts and one, a sugar (placebo) pill. At the end of 12 weeks, the blood level of selenium was increased by 60 percent in both the selenium pill group and the Brazil nut group. The increases in both groups were statistically significant compared to the people taking the placebo pill. The authors concluded that a daily Brazil nut is just as effective as a supplement. Interestingly enough, the average amount of selenium in the two Brazil nuts is half that of the supplement (53 micrograms versus 100 micrograms), yet both groups increased their blood selenium level by the same amount, which just goes to show that a smaller amount of the real food can be just as effective as a larger dose of a supplement. I eat two Brazil nuts in my oatmeal every day, and though the quantity of selenium may vary from nut to nut, I don't feel the need to take any extra selenium in pill form.

And now to the question, is there any scientific evidence that eating foods high in selenium will have a positive effect on the thyroid?

I said above that selenium isn't just important for the thyroid, it is also important for a properly functioning immune system. It is no small wonder that there might be a connection between selenium deficiency and Hashimoto's disease. In fact, in populations living in areas that are deficient in selenium, there is an increased rate of Hashimoto's disease. What I have failed to tell you so far is that Western medicine has not yet found a way to stop the underlying autoimmune process seen in Hashimoto's. Instead, physicians focus on supplementing the declining thyroid hormone levels with either synthetic or natural thyroid hormone.

But what if I were to tell you that there might be a mineral that you could take that could stop the underlying immune process in Hashimoto's disease? I think that would be neat, don't you?

That mineral is selenium. The exciting study that suggested using selenium for Hashimoto's disease was done in Munich, Germany, with 70 female patients with the disease who were randomly placed into two groups. The 36 patients in group one were given 200 micrograms of selenium daily for three months. The 34 patients in the control group received a placebo pill. After three months, the researchers found that in the patients with the highest amount of anti-TPO Ab (see page 45), there was a 40-percent decrease in antibody levels in the patients taking selenium and a 10 percent increase in anti-TPO Ab levels in the patients taking the placebo pill. In fact, nine patients in the selenium-treated group saw their antibody levels drop to those seen in healthy people. When these nine patients' thyroids were examined using ultrasound, their ultrasound patterns had also returned to those seen in normal people!

Though this study is small and the levels of anti-TPO Ab can fluctuate for many reasons, it is thought-provoking. I don't see a down side to eating two Brazil nuts every day to get a little extra selenium. Who knows, it may even prevent you from developing a thyroid problem in the first place!

CORTISOL AND THE ADRENAL GLAND

We all have two adrenal glands that sit on top of the kidneys and make a number of hormones that are important for life. One part of the gland makes a hormone called aldosterone, which is intimately involved with controlling salt levels in the blood and blood pressure. Another part of the gland produces adrenaline, the chemical that surges through our bodies when we are frightened, giving us sweaty palms, a racing heart and butterflies in our stomachs. The adrenal gland also makes cortisol, the hormone that is designed to help us cope with stress.

Let's go back to those happy days when we used to have to hunt for food in a forest rather than in a grocery store.

Picture a Paleolithic man replete with stone spear and ax, trekking through the brush in hot pursuit of a four-legged lunch, which is hopping away as fast as possible. Suddenly there is a rustle in the bushes and the hunter is now face-to-face with a tiger, whose long white teeth glisten in the afternoon sun. Mr. Paleolithic Man promptly turns and flees in the opposite direction in panic, listening to the sounds of paws closing in on him.

In an effort for us all to help our poor ancestor, let's brainstorm for a moment and think about how the tanned and muscular body of our friend can help keep him from the impending doom. In order for him to run, his legs need lots of blood so that his muscles can get plenty of nutrients and oxygen. When he first saw the tiger, he probably broke into a cold sweat. That was caused by his adrenal gland pumping out adrenaline, which immediately diverted blood flow from his skin and gut, and channeled it all to his muscles. That helped him for a while, but if that large, hungry cat doesn't give up so easily, Mr. Paleolithic Man will need to continue to feed his muscles with energy. He won't have time to stop for a snack, so he will have to use his energy stores to keep his blood glucose levels up.

This is where the hormone cortisol comes in. Cortisol stimulates fat and carbohydrate metabolism to make extra sugar in the blood. Of course, we wouldn't want the sugar levels in the blood to get too high, so the cortisol also stimulates the release of insulin from the pancreas, which helps maintain the blood glucose levels in the normal range.

Through the stress hormone cortisol, our caveman cousin can continue to run, climb and hide, with a plentiful supply of energy, in the form of glucose, running through his blood vessels.

The amount of cortisol in your bloodstream is controlled by the pituitary gland, and it doesn't remain constant throughout the day. It is highest just before we wake up in the morning and lowest around midnight, when, hopefully, we are asleep. This up and down variation in cortisol levels can be altered if someone is under chronic stress.

What happens to the body if you are always stressed and your cortisol level is always high? You gain weight! Don't believe me? Have you ever met somebody who had to be put on a high dose of steroid drugs for a long time? Prednisone and the other pharmaceuticals like it are chemical versions of our body's own cortisol. These drugs are lifesaving for many people, but they tend to make them eat ravenously and put on weight. In fact, there is a relatively rare medical condition called Cushing's disease, where a small tumor in the pituitary gland causes the adrenal gland to make far too much cortisol. Patient's with Cushing's disease all become fat, especially in the abdominal area. This abdominal fat is actually the worst type of fat you can have because it is associated with heart attacks and stroke.

Okay, people on steroids or with Cushing's disease get fat, but what happens with normal people who are under stress? Let's look at the some of the evidence and you decide for yourselves!

Two groups of young ladies spent three days in a laboratory doing stressful cognitive tests. One group had 30 healthy but heavy young ladies; the other group had 29 healthy, thin young ladies. The researchers measured blood cortisol levels during these sessions and also performed assessments on the women to gauge their levels of psychological distress. The results were fascinating.

The heavy women felt the laboratory challenges were more threatening, did worse on them and reported more chronic stress compared to the thin ladies. They also made significantly more cortisol on the first day of the tests compared to their thinner counterparts.

Here is the cool part. Some of the heavy women weren't heavy all over, their fat was all centered on their waists, and these women continued to make higher amounts of cortisol on days two and three despite the fact they were familiar with the challenges.

The authors concluded that waist fat is related to greater psychological vulnerability to stress and to higher cortisol levels, and that this supports the hypothesis that stress-induced cortisol secretion contributes to belly fat!

But forget about a fat belly. How about a heart attack? Recent research published in the October 2013 edition of *Journal of the American College of Cardiology* from the University College London showed a frightening new link between elevated cortisol levels in response to stress and signs of damage to the heart muscle. The study was conducted over two years and included over 500 healthy men and women in their 50s, 60s and 70s, all of whom underwent psychological and physiological testing.

What they found when these people were stressed through psychological testing (picture the SATs) was that, not only did the level of cortisol in their saliva increase (not a big surprise as cortisol is the stress hormone), but there was also an increase in blood levels of a substance called troponin, which gets released by the heart muscle when it is being damaged. In fact, elevated troponin levels are one of the ways that your doctor can tell if you are having a heart attack!

So it appears that too much cortisol can make you fat and give you a heart attack. But before you all conclude that your stressful lifestyle is all to blame for those extra inches and chest pains, I must tell you that the relationship between adrenal function, cortisol and weight is very complex. In fact, it is not always easy to predict whether somebody's stress level will result in high cortisol and a beer belly. However, my own opinion is that stress doesn't help, and whether it causes stress eating or abdominal obesity through too much cortisol, no one can successfully lose weight if he or she hasn't found healthy ways to cope with it.

Before we leave the world of cortisol and the wonderful adrenal gland, permit me to say a few words about dietary supplements that are being aggressively marketed on the Internet to lower cortisol levels and help with weight loss. Then I'll tell you about a substance to avoid if you want to keep your cortisol low and your belly lean.

If you were to go to the website MedicineNet.com, part of the Web MD network, you'd find an article titled "Stress, Hormones and Weight Gain," which aptly summarizes the current state of affairs regarding dietary supplements that lower cortisol levels.

"No independent studies published in respected, peer-reviewed medical journals have shown that these supplements have any value in cortisol reduction or weight loss. In fact, exercise is the best method for lowering cortisol levels that have risen in response to stress and has the added benefit of burning calories to stimulate weight loss."

I couldn't have put it better myself. Now to the substance to avoid, salt.

But before I give you the evidence for the link between eating salt and increasing cortisol levels, I do want you to know that salt has got a bad rap just like butter.

You may have recently read in the news that saturated fat, the stuff that butter is made out of, isn't so bad for you. That may well be true. As we discussed in the last chapter, saturated fat isn't an evil, just an annoyance—remember? It's just that, because nuts, seeds, olive and avocado oils are much better for you than the saturated fat found in red meat and full-fat dairy, why spend all your fat calories on butter (a C-grade) fat?

And as for our obsession with all things low-salt. . .

Let's look at the evidence from Swedish researchers, published in the April 2014 edition of the *American Journal of Hypertension*. In this paper, scientists analyzed data from 25 studies and more than 274,000 people and found that eating more than 5 grams of salt per day is associated with a 16-percent increased risk of dying and a 12-percent increased risk of heart disease—all of this is old news.

The surprising thing that they also found is that people who ate between 2.5 and 5 grams of salt per day had a lower risk of dying and developing heart disease compared to the people on the low-salt (less than 2.5 grams per day) diets. So some salt appears to be a good idea after all.

That is good news for your food and for your palate. The problem with salt is that it definitely increases your cortisol levels.

Chilean researchers recruited 370 patients aged 18–85, 60 percent of them having metabolic syndrome (problems with weight, sugar, blood pressure, low good cholesterol, high triglycerides) and looked at the relationship between their salt intake and the cortisol levels in their urine. They found that increased salt intake is associated with increased levels of cortisol in the urine and increased risk of insulin resistance (we will get to insulin momentarily). They even hypothesized that it is the increased cortisol levels "that may partially explain the metabolic disturbances observed with a liberal salt diet." Bottom line—some salt good, more salt not good.

INSULIN AND THE PANCREAS

We finish this section by briefly reviewing what we said in Chapter 1 about insulin, the body's storage hormone, which is designed to store every excess calorie you eat by turning it into fat.

Insulin is produced in the pancreas and helps maintain normal glucose levels in the bloodstream. It makes the blood glucose go down, and glucagon (another hormone made by your pancreas) makes it go up, so that through a delicate balance of these two hormones, your blood glucose levels remain fairly constant throughout the day.

Now just in case you have forgotten, the storage hormone insulin allows sugar in your blood to pass into your cells, where it will either be burned for energy (that is good) or turned into fat for "winter" storage (that is not good). It therefore stands to reason that if insulin promotes fat formation in fat cells, then someone with high insulin levels would find it difficult to lose weight. It is for this reason that I measure the fasting insulin levels of my patients all the time, because if the levels are high, it can help explain some of the weight issues.

Many patients ask me the following question, "If I have high circulating insulin levels, is there anything I can do to get them back to normal?" And I answer, "Of course there is." My diet will drop your insulin levels, and exercise will too! There are also some prescription medications like metformin and Byetta, to name just two, that have been shown in clinical studies to not only drop elevated insulin level but also reduce weight.

For those of you who are reluctant to take drugs, there is also a mineral that has been shown in a clinical study to lower fasting insulin levels. Chromium is a naturally occurring, steely-gray, hard metal that is required by the body in trace amounts for both sugar and cholesterol metabolism. The recommended daily amount of chromium according to the National Academy of Sciences is 25–35 mcg. Want to eat a food that will give you all the chromium that you need for the day? Try a cup of broccoli.

A clinical study of 26 healthy young men used a much higher dose of chromium, more than 220 mcg per day, for three months. The results showed that in the individuals with the highest fasting insulin levels, taking chromium led to a statistically significant decrease in fasting insulin levels.

In closing this chapter, I hope you will agree that many different hormones in your body have a great influence on your ability to lose weight, lower your fasting blood glucose and drop your cholesterol. I also hope that I have given you some strategies to help keep your hormone levels optimal and therefore allow you to reap the benefits of all your efforts.

3

THE "MONEY"

WHAT EXACTLY TO EAT AND WHY

We are finally here, the part where I tell you exactly what to eat and why. You are probably asking yourself at this point, "Why did it take so many pages to get to the details?"

You're right! This book could be much simpler and shorter. I could have opened by just telling you what to eat and why, and you would have been on your way.

You are not alone! Many of the patients I see are eager to start this diet and are disappointed when I begin by ordering labs and talking about starch, sugar and saturated fat instead of explaining the specifics of their new eating plan. So why did I beat around the bush?

Since we know each other a little better now, I think it is about time I reiterated two important facts about my clinical practice. The first is that I see more patients for weight loss, diabetes and cholesterol issues than for all other conditions combined. So I deal with these issues every day. The second fact is that I have had a lot of success with my dietary approach. Patients are referred to me by every type of physician from all over the New York, New Jersey and Connecticut areas for weight loss, cholesterol and blood glucose problems. So I need you to put your trust in me, as there is a method to my madness.

Again, the reason is simple. As I said before, if you don't ensure the foundation is strong, the house will crumble at the first sign of stress.

Starting my dietary approach when we haven't done all our homework and ascertained why other diets haven't worked is a recipe for temporary success but eventual failure. As I said in the last chapter, no one can lose weight if his hormones are off, so if we don't identify and treat those hormonal issues, you won't lose a pound even if you eat like a saint.

I also want to tell you that no one can lose weight when he's depressed. So you need to understand and recognize that, if you have a tendency to stress eat with comfort food and you don't deal with this issue (we will talk about this in Chapter 4), you may lose ten pounds (4.5 kg), but the moment the day goes badly, you will spiral downward into despair at your local frozen yogurt place.

Now we have done our due diligence. Let's begin.

In this chapter we'll go over the foods you'll enjoy for breakfast, lunch and dinner, and the three snacks you must eat in between. I'll also talk about why these particular foods were chosen and go over the research behind their health benefits in general and cholesterol-, weight- and sugar-lowering properties in particular.

HERE IS THE DIET IN A NUTSHELL

Breakfast is Bran Buds or SmartBran, a yogi yogurt bowl or frittata (you'll learn all about these and other recipes in the very next chapter, so definitely read on).

Lunch is a lean protein like salmon or steak, pork-and-bean stew and other varied delights from Gavin's kitchen.

Dinner is another type of lean protein, such as chicken oreganata or enchilada or even old-time scrambled eggs or crustless quiche.

A midmorning fruit snack and a midafternoon fruit snack in between meals, an 85-percent dark chocolate square to be sucked liked a lozenge, and a handful of nuts round off the menu.

If you want to switch things around and have the nuts and chocolate later on after an early dinner, then you can. As long as we are keeping to eating six times per day, every two to three hours, we are good to go.

That's all, folks. Now let's go do it!

BREAKFAST—NEVER AGAIN A DOUGHNUT!

Most people have their last meal of the day at seven or eight o'clock at night and sit down to breakfast between six thirty and seven thirty the following morning. If you do the math, you'll realize that you may not eat anything for almost 12 hours of the day. Your body easily adapts to this daily fast, but in order to keep things running smoothly, it will require sustenance upon waking in order to break the fast. That is where the word breakfast comes from, and the purpose of breakfast is to break the fasting state that we enter every night.

You have to eat breakfast. It is not optional. Here's why:

The Man Diet is about 1,000–1,100 calories per day. One of the many neat things about this eating plan is that you will eat less, more often. You'll have three meals and three snacks per day. You'll eat every two to three hours, and those around you will probably notice that you're always eating. What the bystanders should appreciate is not *that* you are eating but *what* you are eating.

If you miss a snack or meal and go four to five hours during the day without eating something, you will become famished. Don't let that happen. Hungry people are not happy people. Unhappy people make bad food choices.

A balanced breakfast has all the three major food groups we know and love so well, adequately represented. There are many ways to achieve this, but if you want to lower your cholesterol, you have to be much more discerning about your breakfast choices.

When I introduced you to the carbohydrate family at the beginning of the book, I talked about fiber. Fiber is a complex carbohydrate that the body cannot digest and turn into glucose. Fiber is good for you, as a recent 500,000-person study sponsored by the National Institutes of Health demonstrated. The study showed that people who ate more than 25–30 grams of fiber per day had a 22 percent lower risk of dying from any cause over a nine-year period compared to those who ate only small amounts of fiber every day.

However, we have to be even more discerning than simply having a high-fiber breakfast if we want the real magic to happen. There are two different types of fiber, soluble and insoluble. Most people choose the high-fiber cereals that are made from wheat bran, which is an insoluble fiber. Those are great, but the advantage of eating cereals that are high in soluble fiber is that the soluble fiber also lowers your cholesterol. So instead of wheat bran, look for products that are made predominantly from oats or psyllium.

Now for the specifics, so you know exactly what and more importantly what not to put in your mouth.

Let's start off with a great cereal made by Nature's Path called SmartBran. It is packed with 13 grams of fiber (some of which is soluble) and also has 3 grams of protein per serving. The serving size is two-thirds of a cup (20 g), and the cereal is high in both psyllium and oats for that double soluble fiber whammy. You can find this at many stores or online.

Another option is Kellogg's All-Bran Buds, which also contains 13 grams of fiber and is made with psyllium husks. It too has 3 grams of protein. The recommended portion size is one-third of a cup (10 g), which doesn't sound like a lot until you feel it sitting in your stomach. You'll be full, I assure you!

I do realize that All-Bran Buds is mass-produced and contains sugar. I prefer the SmartBran, which has evaporated cane juice instead. However, the purpose of writing this book is for you to be able to keep my diet wherever you live, and so I feel it is important to recommend products that are available in your local grocery store.

Many patients ask me about Multi Grain Cheerios, which is made from oats. Below is some of the information on the nutrition label for Multi Grain Cheerios. We have already learned how to read a nutrition label in Chapter 1, where we also learned to watch out for those sneaky starches that aren't listed on the label.

Let's look at the label together and decide for ourselves what we think of this famed breakfast cereal.

NUTRITION FACTS SERVING SIZE—1 CUP (29 G)	
CALORIES 110—CALORIES FROM FAT 10	
TOTAL FAT	1 g
SAT. FAT	0 g
TRANS FAT	0 g
POLYUNSATURATED FAT	0.5 g
CHOLESTEROL	0 mg
SODIUM	120 mg
TOTAL CARBS.	24 g
DIETARY FIBER	3 g
SUGARS	6 g
OTHER CARBOHYDRATE	15 g
PROTEIN	2 g

For your 110-calorie breakfast, you get 24 grams of total carbohydrates, and 3 grams of that is any type of fiber.

Now, simple math will tell you that 24 - 3 = 21, so you are getting 21 grams of nonfiber, or net carbohydrates, per serving. Of those 21 grams, 6 grams are clearly listed as sugars, so there is a hidden 15 grams of starch that you can see only if you read between the lines and can count!

SmartBran and All-Bran Buds both contain 24 grams of total carbohydrates, but a whopping 13 grams of that total is made up of soluble and insoluble fiber. There is, therefore, only about 11 grams per serving of nonfiber, or net carbohydrates. Of those 11 grams, 6 grams come from sugars, so there is a hidden 5 grams of starch in these two products.

The simple truth is that Multi Grain Cheerios has too little fiber and too much hidden starch, compared to the other two cereals, so I don't recommend it.

Even our friendly oatmeal doesn't compete with these two fiber-packed cereals. Oatmeal is okay, though it has about 15 grams of net carbs and should therefore not be your main cereal of choice. If you do have a yen for it sometimes, eat about 4–6 ounces (113.5–170 g) of plain cooked oatmeal sprinkled with a teaspoon of cinnamon on top. If you use instant, just remember that under no circumstances should you buy any of the flavored varieties. You should flavor all oatmeal yourself with cinnamon or a teaspoon of honey instead.

Let me take this opportunity to tell you another simple rule to live by: Never buy food that has already been flavored or sweetened. If you want to sweeten or flavor something, do it yourself with a couple of berries, cinnamon or a drop of honey. Gone are the days of purchasing food that has been flavored and sweetened by some multinational food company and is therefore packed with sugar, high-fructose corn syrup or who knows what else.

We are almost done with breakfast. Two more points and you can begin to eat!

First, you may want to use some form of milk with your cereal. Certain people have digestive and other problems with cow or soy milk, so I recommend almond milk as a refreshing and new taste to go along with your new healthy cereal. If this is not to your liking, then soy or low-fat (1%) cow's milk are acceptable alternatives for some people.

Second, I would like you to sprinkle two teaspoons (10 g) of ground flaxseed on your cereal every day. Flax is another soluble fiber and is also high in omega-3 fatty acids, which help lower inflammation and triglyceride levels. Store the packet in the fridge after you open it to keep it fresh and prevent those wonderful omega-3 oils from going rancid. By the way, with all that extra fiber you will now be consuming, your bowel movements will be abundant!

LUNCH AND DINNER—VARIATIONS ON A THEME

Lunch and dinner consist of a lean protein served on a bed of fresh salad for lunch and on an assortment of colorful vegetables for dinner. Sound charming?

The proteins are all lean, which means that they are not packed with lots of saturated fat. There are five basic protein groups that you can choose from. You definitely want to vary the proteins so that you don't get bored. In other words, if you eat a protein from one group for lunch, pick a different protein from another group for dinner. Since there are five protein groups, and you have seven lunches and seven dinners to cater for yourself, you'll find that you eat from each protein group two to three times per week. Whatever you do, don't eat chicken for every meal; you will rapidly find this diet awfully dull, and then it will all be over with a cluck!

Here are the five groups, together with some of the latest research showing how these foods are so good for you.

THE FAMOUS DIET FOODS: LEAN MEAT AND POULTRY

Protein group number one is the most obvious one, poultry and lean red meat. You can eat any of the following: skinless chicken breast, skinless turkey breast, pork tenderloin, buffalo, bison, ostrich or extra-lean beef (five cuts of the cow are extra lean). To be clear and at the risk of sounding like a dictator, the list above is the only meat products you can enjoy at this stage. Any other type of meat is off limits until we get your weight, cholesterol and blood glucose down. To put it another way: If it is not on the list, it is not going in!

Here is the research so you can see why this works:

A Harvard study published in 2010 based on 84,000 women over a 26-year period showed that replacing daily beef, pork or lamb with chicken or turkey lowered these ladies' risk of heart disease by 19 percent.

Other important substitutions were a 30-percent reduction if you swapped those daily meats for nuts, a 24-percent reduction if you swapped them for fish, and a 13-percent reduction if you swapped them for low-fat dairy.

It will therefore come as no great shock for you to learn that fish is protein group number two, and low-fat dairy rounds off our list as protein group number five. You'll have to wait until the snack chapter to go nuts about nuts!

How much can I eat at each meal is the next obvious question.

The answer is that the amount of protein you need every day varies with how big you are. Clearly, if you are 6 feet 6 inches (2 m) and 250 pounds (113 kg), you will have a larger frame and higher daily protein needs than if you are a slight 5 feet 2 inches (1.6 m) and weigh 150 pounds (68 kg). I therefore recommend that a serving size of protein at each meal is approximately the size of the palm of your hand. This could be anywhere from 4 to 7 ounces (198 g), depending upon how large your hand is. Large people tend to have larger hands, and the smaller among us have more diminutive palms. Don't go crazy and start measuring and weighing things. You can estimate, and if you take a little extra, it is not the end of the world for the reasons that we will now discuss.

For years, various diet gurus have said that eating lots of protein helps weight loss. For example, the Atkins diet substitutes protein for carbohydrate. However, many nutritionists voice concern about these high-protein fads, worrying that all that extra protein will cause strain on the liver and kidneys.

Thomas Halton and Frank Hu from the Department of Nutrition at Harvard Medical School wrote a review paper on the subject, which appeared in the Journal of the American College of Nutrition in 2004. I'll highlight the key points:

"There is convincing evidence that a higher protein intake increases thermogenesis . . . compared to diets of lower protein content."

Increases what? I hear you exclaim.

"Increases thermogenesis," the article said.

Thermogenesis is the amount of energy the body needs to digest, use and dispose of different types of food.

Because of the chemical composition of protein, the body has to work harder to process and utilize this food compared to carbohydrates. Approximately 20 to 35 percent of the calories you get from eating protein will be burned up by your body just to process the stuff. Carbohydrates are a more efficient and cleaner fuel, as only 5 to 15 percent of their calories is needed to digest and metabolize them. Using a less-efficient fuel in your car means that you fill up at the gas station more often. That is bad if you are trying to save money on gas, but good if you are trying to lose weight. By eating more protein and less carbohydrates, you are substituting a less-efficient fuel with a more efficient one. More of the calories you eat are being burned up by your metabolism, and you will lose weight.

"There is convincing evidence that a higher protein intake increases satiety . . . compared to diets of lower protein content."

Satiety is the feeling of fullness after a meal. Multiple experiments on healthy people have shown that eating a high-protein meal makes the subject feel fuller and less desirous of eating again compared to when they eat a meal lower in protein.

"There is evidence that higher protein intakes can significantly increase the risk of kidney stones."

You better believe it! I have seen two patients in the last few weeks who both told me that they had lost pounds and pounds on the Atkins diet only to end up in the emergency room with kidney stones and childbirth-like cramps.

"There is little evidence that high-protein diets pose a serious risk to kidney function in healthy populations. More susceptible groups such as diabetics and those with existing renal [kidney] disease should exercise more caution with higher protein intakes."

The bottom line is that I have no issue with being a little more generous with your protein serving as it may help you lose weight and keep you less hungry. However, unlimited protein could put you in the hospital with kidney stones, and if you have any kidney issues or are diabetic, then a high-protein diet isn't for you. Lucky for all of us, my diet isn't high in protein, and the proteins you do eat are all the good ones to boot!

FISH AND SEAFOOD

Protein source number two comes from the water. You can eat any fish or seafood you like except the following four: no lobster, shrimp, octopus or calamari. They are all too high in cholesterol and should be avoided for the time being. You should also take care with fish that are high in mercury, like swordfish. The Environmental Protection Agency has a list of fish with the highest mercury levels on its website, so take a look at that before you stock up. The serving size for fish is exactly the same as it is for poultry and lean meat—the palm of your hand.

By now, you are probably asking yourself the following important question: "How do I cook these proteins that I will eat for lunch and dinner?"

You can cook the protein any way you want—sauté, bake, grill, boil, broil or roast. You can use avocado oil as your main cooking oil of choice—it is packed with healthy fats and is very stable at high temperatures. If you aren't cooking but are just adding oil and spices to a salad, I particularly favor olive oil for the health reasons that we will see in a few moments.

The one thing you can't do is fry anything. Any other cooking method is acceptable.

Why no frying, you ask with a tearful sob.

I'll answer that by taking another look at a famous study. *The Women's Health Initiative* was the government-funded study that showed an increased risk of breast cancer and heart disease in women who took hormone replacement therapy after menopause. This study looked at lots of other things, including diet. The study's researchers reported in May 2011 that women eating baked or broiled fish five times per week had a 30 percent lower risk of heart failure compared to those who ate fish less than once per week. They also found that consuming fried fish at least once per week was associated with a 48 percent increased risk of heart failure.

PULSES—ALSO KNOWN AS BEANS TO THE REST OF US

The third protein source is beans. All beans are good. They are a little starchy, so I recommend eating them only a couple of times per week. You can mix beans with ground chicken breast or ground turkey breast and make a curry or a chili if you like. As long as you stick to the approximately palm-size serving with each meal, you are good to go. If you are a vegetarian or vegan, this group will be your main protein source, though under those circumstances you might also like to investigate a fungal protein called Quorn or even seitan (the protein found in wheat, aka gluten, as in what many people avoid in their gluten-free diets). I recommend all this in an effort to mix things up a little and widen your more restricted protein options.

I personally like tofu, or bean curd, which is made from fermented soybean milk. It is featured heavily in Asian cuisine. Some people can be allergic to soy or find that they have problems digesting it. In that case, you still have many other bean options available, though soy is one of the only plant proteins that contains all the essential amino acids that we need to get from our food (other proteins with those eight essential amino acids include spirulina, derived from algae and hemp protein, which comes from the cannabis plant). If you find that too many beans make you bloated or gaseous, then some digestive enzymes with meals, easily purchased at any health food store, will help keep the gas down and the belly less bloated.

Ready for the study on soy protein, milk protein and blood pressure? This one came out in August 2011.

Researchers from Tulane University in New Orleans took 352 adults with mildly elevated blood pressure and gave them 40 grams of milk protein as a powder every day for eight weeks, asking them not to alter their total calories or exercise level during the same period. The researchers waited a few weeks and did the same for another eight weeks with the same people, this time using 40 grams of soy protein powder instead of the milk protein. Finally, after waiting yet another few weeks, they gave the participants a powder that contained 40 grams of carbohydrates for a final eight weeks.

And the results are in!

Using the soy or milk protein powder significantly dropped the blood pressure by 2 mmHg. Now, that doesn't sound very impressive until you realize that dropping your blood pressure by 2 mmHg lowers your risk of having a stroke by 6 percent, which is a little more significant. The soy protein powder also significantly increased the good cholesterol (HDL) levels too. Just another good reason to love tofu, wouldn't you say?

It will come as no great shock to you to learn that adding an extra 40 grams of carbohydrate did nothing to help the blood pressure or the cholesterol. I think these people were lucky that they got only eight weeks of the sugary powder. Any longer and they would have started to see some real problems, I am sure.

EGGS, THE BREAKFAST OF CHAMPIONS

Eggs are a fourth protein source. Three egg whites as an omelet with cooked vegetables is a great meal option. If you want, you can even add a single yolk into the mix to get a little yellow onto the canvas. An egg white salad with low-fat mayonnaise is another option to entertain. Also, if you are getting sick of the daily cereal for breakfast, you can always try a couple of egg whites from time to time with mushrooms and sautéed onions. Just remember that you don't want to eat egg whites every day. There are plenty of other protein options. As I said above, you must vary and rotate your proteins so that your palate doesn't get bored.

DAIRY—LOW FAT OR DEATH!

If you don't have any milk issues, then low-fat dairy is a fifth healthy protein option on your list. All the cheese you eat must be low fat. If the product doesn't expressly state that it is low or reduced in fat, then it isn't, and you cannot put it in your mouth. Low-fat cheeses are now all the rage, and you can find lots of new varieties and flavors, so explore the dairy aisle. It will be quite an experience!

If the low-fat cheeses appear a little waxlike, you can improve their general texture by cooking them. For example, try adding a little low-fat grated cheese to an egg white omelet. Two to three ounces (57–85 g) of low-fat cheese will give you more than 20 grams of protein and can happily crown a fresh garden salad for a light and healthy lunch. Yogurt and cottage cheese are also great options, as long as they are low fat too.

Just to remind you again about flavoring and sweetening: all the yogurt you buy should be plain. You flavor everything yourself with fresh berries, vanilla essence or a drop of honey. Never buy flavored yogurt again! It contains lots of sugar or an artificial sweetener, and as I am not even sure what that goo at the bottom of the container actually is, it isn't going in either your mouth or mine!

The next question we must ask ourselves is, What can we eat with this lean protein?

For lunch you can enjoy your lean and healthy protein on a bed of salad. And yes, you can have as much salad as you like. Just to clarify, a salad contains things like lettuce, cabbage, tomatoes, spinach, cucumbers, pepper, and so on. Vegetables slathered in mayonnaise is not a salad, so coleslaw is out. On top of the salad and protein, feel free to pour a low-fat or low-sugar dressing, balsamic vinegar or olive oil to make things more exotic. You can even sprinkle some seeds on top of the salad, but dried berries are out as they are too high in sugar. I love olive oil and prefer to bathe salads in that light yellow liquid. You can use a teaspoon or even a little more if you would like. A study from June 2011 by the University of Bordeaux, France, found that in the more than 7,000 older people who were observed for more than five years, those who consumed the highest amount of olive oil in their dressings and food had a 41 percent lower stroke rate compared to those who didn't use olive oil at all, proving that it is all good when it comes to olive oil.

For dinner choose another type of lean protein that will be eaten on a bed of vegetables, such as sprouts, cauliflower, a few turnips or carrots, string beans and so on. These vegetables are generally starchier, so I prefer that you have a light salad for lunch with the heavier, denser vegetables saved for the evening repast. Again, you can cook these vegetables however you like, as long as you don't go crazy and deep-fry them.

On a more humorous note, my most amusing patient asked me if she had to literally lie on a bed of vegetables when eating dinner! I replied that, "It is the protein, my dear, that is lying on top of the bed vegetables. I have no preference as to where you dine or of what your linens are made!"

Wait a minute . . .

Salad for lunch and vegetables for dinner? How can I be so cruel?

The reason is that I want you to stay alive, and all those vegetables are going to help you do just that. We now go to Oxford University in merry old England to see what I mean. In January 2011, researchers published the results of a huge population study called *EPIC*, which included more than 300,000 people from ten different countries. The bottom line of the study was that the people who ate eight or more servings of fruit and veggies every day had a 22 percent reduction in the risk of dying from heart disease compared to those who didn't eat a lot of fruit and vegetables.

Just to clear things up, a single serving of salad is about the same size as a baseball, and a serving of the more starchy evening vegetable like broccoli is about the size of a scoop of ice cream. On your new and delicious diet you'll easily eat five to six servings of veggies per day. We haven't yet talked about snacks, but you'll soon see that two pieces of fruit per day are also on the menu. Therefore, following my diet will not only provide you with a lot of fruit and vegetables, but it will also, apparently, reduce your risk of dying of a massive heart attack. Not a bad deal really when you think about it.

We are about to learn what our three daily snack options are and what beverages we may use to refresh our parched palates. Before we do that, however, let me state the obvious:

I have spent the last few pages telling you what to eat. Permit me now to give you the list of the foods that are not to enter your mouth. You are not to eat the staples of the world that we talked about in Chapter 1. There is no bread of any kind, no rice, no pasta, no potatoes, not even yams or sweet potatoes. There is also no corn, quinoa, teff, buckwheat or any other kind of starch-filled grain. Your only grains are the soluble fiber ones, psyllium and oats, which you have been enjoying for your daily breakfast.

You look shocked and upset. How can you live without bread or another of those starchy staples? Just remember two things:

This diet is not forever. It is designed to help you lose weight and drop your cholesterol and blood glucose. It will turn your body back into what it was always supposed to be. You will eat bread again if you want to, just not now.

At this stage, I should explain to you that there are really two phases to this diet. The first one is designed to get your weight back to its optimal level and at the same time lower your cholesterol and blood glucose numbers so that you are no longer a candidate for prescription medications. Once we have achieved these lofty but attainable goals, we will shift to phase two, which is where you decide how you want to eat from now on. This part is more individualized, and I'll explain all about it in great detail in the final chapter of this book. For now, just rely on the fact that you will see high-quality starches back on the menu eventually, if you so wish!

I have used this dietary approach with thousands upon thousands of people, and now two clinical trials using this diet have been published, proving its effectiveness. It is totally safe, and people usually feel great after the first few grumpy days. Many patients report that they feel less heavy and bloated, more energized and even excited as they watch their waistlines shrink.

I know the idea of no starch sounds hard, but you can do this, I promise.

SNACKS—BE A HAPPY SNACKER!

You are going to eat two pieces of fruit every day, one as a midmorning snack and one as a midafternoon snack. The fruits you can eat are all low (less than 50) on the glycemic index (which we now know all about) and won't cause your blood glucose levels to soar and plummet like a fishing boat in a stormy sea. Behold our new favorite fruits: apples, pears, bananas, cherries, peaches, plums, apricots (not dried), oranges and grapefruit. You may substitute one of your fruit snacks for a handful of berries. In a moment we shall describe just how good berries are for your health, but first two caveats. The first is that, although I told you that you could enjoy two fruit snacks every day, one of the snacks must be an apple or a pear. The reason for this is simple: they contain high amounts of a soluble fiber called pectin. As we already know, soluble fiber makes your cholesterol go down, so enjoy your daily apple or pear. Caveat number two is about bananas. This delicious yellow fruit can get quite high in sugar if it gets too soft, so I recommend you stick to the harder variety.

Many of my patients routinely ask me about their favorite fruit snacks that do not appear on the permitted list, so let me briefly share with you the higher glycemic index fruit that are to be avoided for the time being: mangoes, raisins, dried apricots, watermelon, papaya, cantaloupe and pineapple, to name but a few of these sweeter fruits. All the fruit delicacies just mentioned score greater than 50 on the glycemic index, and I would prefer that you stick to two daily fruit snacks from their less sugary cousins.

ALL HAIL THE HUMBLE BERRY!

Berries are spectacular foods. They are low on the glycemic index and are packed with antioxidants, which are naturally occurring substances that can protect your body from the disease-causing effects of dangerous molecules called free radicals that are produced by the body's own metabolism. Each color and hue of a berry is a different pigment that can have multiple health-promoting activities. Let me illustrate the point for you.

In April 2011, Xiang Gao, MD, PhD, and his colleagues from Harvard reported the results of a 130,000-person study at the American Academy of Neurology's annual meeting. His group found that the men and women who consumed the highest amounts of anthocyanins—a flavonoid antioxidant found in berries, had a 22 percent reduction in the risk of developing Parkinson's disease. Anthocyanins are dark purple-blue pigments and are found in abundance in acai berries, black currants, blackberries and blueberries. So berries are good, and you should feel free to enjoy them in moderation. Half a cup (75 g) is a reasonable serving size; a bucketful would be eating to excess.

ORGANIC OR NOT ORGANIC, THAT IS THE QUESTION

Did you know that some pesticides have now been found to contain chemicals that promote obesity? On May 11, 2010, the White House Task Force on Childhood Obesity released a report called *Solving the Problem of Childhood Obesity Within a Generation*. In the report, the task force listed endocrine-disrupting chemicals (EDCs) as a possible contributing reason for the increased obesity in the country. Some of these EDCs are structurally similar to estrogen and are believed to promote obesity by interfering with the body's own endocrine system, which helps control weight. Here is the kicker. Many of the common pesticides that are sprayed with reckless abandon on our berries, fruit and vegetables are EDCs!

Now for the good news.

Not all produce contains high levels of pesticide. An organization called the Environmental Working Group has come up with a dirty dozen, a list of twelve products with the highest amount of pesticide residue in them. This list can help us work out which organic produce to buy and where we can save money and buy the regular cheap stuff.

Drum roll, please.

Top of the list of dirtiest veggie is the famous diet food, celery. You know, the green sticklike thing that they say takes more calories to chew than you get from eating the stuff? This is followed by peaches, strawberries, apples, blueberries, nectarines, peppers, spinach, kale, cherries, potatoes (which you weren't eating anyway) and grapes (you can have a few grapes from time to time). If you want to go organic, buy the organic option for any of the dirty dozen. Going totally organic is fine but costly and probably unnecessary for such delicacies as onions, avocados, peas, asparagus, cabbage or grapefruit, which all have low pesticide residue anyway. (There are some benefits to going completely organic; they just aren't as pronounced as you might think.)

In 2012, researchers at Stanford reviewed 17 studies in humans and 223 studies of nutrient and contaminant levels in foods to see if organic food was any healthier than conventionally produced products. They found that in the human studies, there was no less chance of developing allergies, asthma, hay fever or food poisoning if people ate only organic. However, they did find that in the studies where they analyzed the nutrient content of organic food, there were definitely fewer pesticides and antibiotics.

My take on this is that, if we are trying to get healthier, then pesticides and antibiotics that will kill the friendly bacteria in our gut are not the way to go. So as I said before, getting the organic version of the dirty dozen seems sensible to me.

Wait a minute. Didn't I say at the beginning of this chapter that you were going to enjoy three snacks per day? Well, aren't we missing another snack? This is the part of the diet where my patients' eyes light up in hopeful expectation. Yes, my friends, there is another snack, and it is a good one.

At about 5 or 6 p.m. you will enjoy a piece of 70 to 85 percent dark chocolate and a handful (20 or so) of unsalted pistachios, almonds or walnuts.

Seriously. I am feeding you chocolate!

Chocolate is another incredible food that contains natural versions of serotonin, adrenaline and even opium. Chocolate is good for your heart, literally. A nine-year study of over 32,000 middle-aged Swedish women found that eating one to three servings per month of chocolate with a high cocoa content (like the 85 percent listed above), reduced their risk of heart failure by 26 percent compared to those who didn't eat the candy at all.

Again, we are talking about a square of 70 to 85 percent dark chocolate every day, which I want you to suck as if it were a lozenge. If you don't like dark chocolate or find the taste not to your liking, increase the quantity of nuts that you eat for your late afternoon snack. Whatever you do, don't substitute the lousy milk chocolate, which is barely a food at all, for the healthy dark chocolate, which is really a medicinal food.

NUTS, BEVERAGES AND BOOZE, AND THEN WE ARE DONE!

Nuts are packed with healthy monounsaturated fats, and they have fiber and protein to boot! I particularly recommend almonds because they contain soluble fiber; pistachios because they have plant cholesterol, which helps you stop absorbing the animal cholesterol you may eat with it; and walnuts, which are high in plant omega-3 fatty acids. Better still, nuts can reverse metabolic syndrome.

In 2008, researchers from Spain divided 1,487 middle-aged and elderly men and women into three groups. The first group was placed on a traditional Mediterranean diet, enriched with a liter of extra virgin olive oil every week. The second group was also put on a Mediterranean diet, but instead of olive oil, they were given an extra 30 grams of mixed nuts every day. The third group was given some general advice on reducing fat in their diet and was the control group. At the start of the study, 60 percent of the people in each group had metabolic syndrome. Let's look at what happened at the end of the study a year later. The percentage of people with metabolic syndrome decreased by 14 percent in the nut group, 7 percent in the olive oil group and only 2 percent in the control group. That is more than a sixfold greater resolution of the metabolic syndrome compared with the control group. Not bad for a bunch of small, hard, roundish things.

The rules on drinks are simple. Water is good, and coffee and tea are okay, as long as you are not overdosing on the caffeine in the vain hopes of boosting your metabolism and losing weight. Regular soda and fruit juices are basically just sugar and therefore not on the list at all, and if they are not on the list, they are not going in. Last but certainly not least is alcohol, which "gladdens the heart of men," as the good book says.

Here's the deal. However much you are drinking, cut it by 50 percent and we'll save some liquid calories. Just remember that some drinking is good for you. I'll prove the point by going back to the EPIC study we met earlier in the chapter. You remember, that massive study conducted in ten European countries?

One of the countries was Greece, and when the Harvard researchers analyzed the Greek data, they found a surprising thing. Moderate alcohol intake (mostly wine) was the single biggest contributor to the longevity seen with the Mediterranean diet. Wine makes you live longer—isn't that terrific! But how much is too much? I hear you ask. To answer, permit me to quote Dr. Dimitrios Trichopoulos, the lead investigator of the study: "My advice to people is to drink wine unless you like it too much." Got it? Good!

BREAKFAST

Simple, quick and easy is the best way to kick off the morning! These delicious starters will help you break your fast without a hitch and send you on your way to a successful, high-energy day!

(ARE YOU KIDDIN' ME!) CRUSTLESS QUICHE

Rich in protein and chock full of garden fresh vegetables, this colorful one-pot breakfast can be eaten hot or cold. Cook once and keep in the fridge for an easy morning grab when you're on the go!

YIELD: 1 QUICHE | SERVINGS: 6 SLICES | SERVING SIZE: 1 SLICE + ⅓ CUP (225 G) SAUCE

---

3 whole eggs

10 egg whites

¼ cup (59 ml) low-fat milk (1% or fat-free)

2 tbsp (30 ml) extra virgin olive oil

½ tsp sea salt (optional)

½ tsp ground black pepper

½ cup (57 g) shredded reduced-fat provolone cheese

½ cup (92 g) cannellini beans, no salt added, drained, rinsed

⅓ cup (50 g) yellow onion, peeled, chopped small

⅓ cup (60 g) red bell pepper, seeded, chopped small

⅓ cup (23 g) broccoli florets, chopped small

¼ cup (25 g) scallion, green and white parts, sliced thin

1 garlic clove, peeled, minced

2 tbsp (5 g) fresh Italian parsley leaves, chopped

2 cup (471 ml) all-natural, low-sodium marinara sauce

Lightly spray or oil the inside surface of a 9-inch (23-cm) glass pie plate. Set aside until needed.

Preheat the oven to 350°F (180°C). Place the oven rack in the center.

In a large bowl, whisk the whole eggs, egg whites, milk, olive oil, salt (optional) and black pepper together until combined. Fold in the cheese, beans, vegetables and herbs.

Pour the mixture into the oiled pie plate. Place in the oven on the center rack and bake for 35–40 minutes or until the center of the quiche is set and no liquid remains when a knife blade is inserted into the center (it should come out clean).

Remove the quiche from the oven and allow it to cool for 5 minutes before serving.

Allow quiche to cool completely before refrigerating, covered, until ready to use. When ready, serve each slice of quiche with cold or warmed marinara sauce.

NUTRITION (PER SERVING)
Calories 220, Total Fat 12 g, Saturated Fat 2.5 g, Trans Fat 0 g, Cholesterol 100 mg, Sodium 300 mg, Total Carbohydrate 12 g, Dietary Fiber 2 g, Sugars 5 g, Protein 15 g, Vitamin A 20%, Vitamin C 35%, Calcium 15%, Iron 10%

TIPS: This is an easy dish to make ahead that can be kept in the refrigerator and used as needed.

Vary the herbs (cilantro leaves, Italian parsley leaves, basil, thyme, rosemary), cheeses (mozzarella, cheddar, feta), beans (black beans, red beans, black eyed peas) and vegetables (chopped spinach, zucchini, tomato).

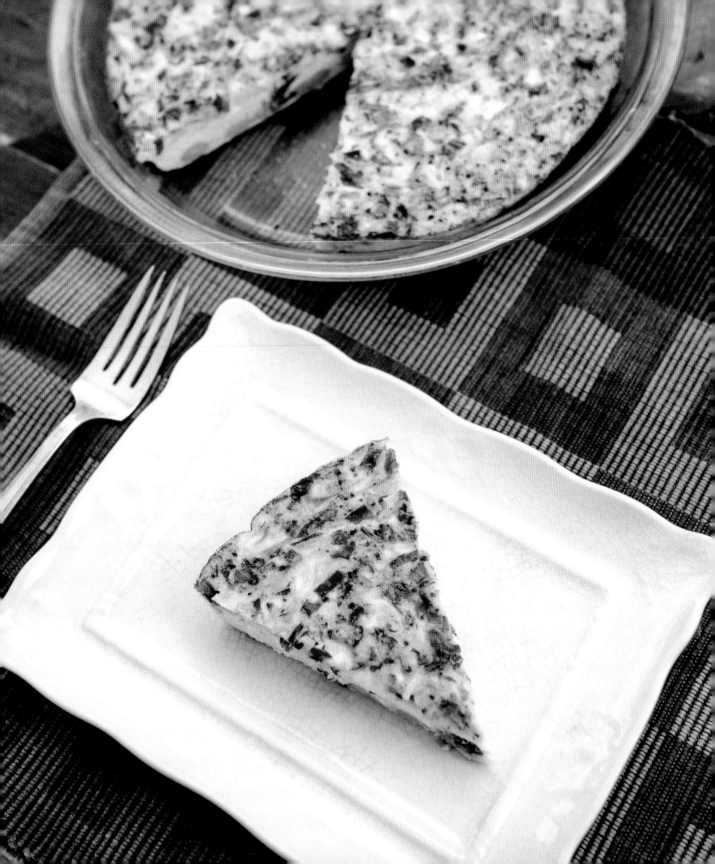

1-2-3 SCRAMBLE

Who says there's no time for breakfast? Soft and cheesy, this high-speed scramble is perfect for a warm and satisfying start to any day! It's as easy as 1-2-3!

YIELD: 1 SCRAMBLE | SERVINGS: 1 | SERVING SIZE: 1 SCRAMBLE

---

1 whole egg

2 egg whites

2 tbsp (30 ml) low-fat milk
(1% or fat-free)

Dash sea salt (optional)

Dash ground black pepper

1 tsp avocado oil

⅓ cup (65 g) tomatoes, diced

½ cup (113 g) baby spinach, chopped

¼ cup (44 g) yellow bell pepper,
seeded, small diced

1 tbsp (3 g) fresh cilantro, chopped

Dash fresh lemon juice

2 tbsp (13 g) reduced-fat shredded
cheddar cheese

Whisk the whole egg, egg whites, milk, salt (optional) and black pepper together and set aside.

Lightly coat the bottom of a small skillet with the oil.

Over medium heat, lightly cook the tomato, spinach and yellow pepper until just tender, about 2 minutes.

Add the egg mixture, cilantro, lemon juice and cheese. Cook, moving the eggs frequently with a spatula until the eggs are firm and moist, but not hard, about 3 minutes.

NUTRITION (PER SERVING)

Calories 230, Total Fat 13 g, Saturated Fat 4 g, Trans Fat 0 g, Cholesterol 195 mg, Sodium 310 mg, Total Carbohydrate 9 g, Dietary Fiber 2 g, Sugars 4 g, Protein 20 g, Vitamin A 50%, Vitamin C 160%, Calcium 25%, Iron 10%

TIPS: Micro Scramble: This dish can be made even quicker in the microwave. Add all the ingredients into a microwave-safe bowl, and cook for 2–3 minutes or until the eggs are firm and moist but not hard.

Vary the fresh chopped herbs (oregano, basil, thyme).

Vary the vegetables (broccoli, artichokes, garlic, red chili flakes, scallions, onion, arugula, zucchini, carrots, mushrooms).

Chop small for quickest cooking.

This is a great place to use up your precooked and leftover vegetables (grilled, roasted, sautéed). Just warm them up in the pan but without the added oil.

HUEVOS RANCHEROS

South of the border flavors star in this traditional morning meal. It'll become a starter staple on your breakfast menu, no matter where you're from!

YIELD: 2 | SERVINGS: 2 | SERVING SIZE: 1

---

1 tsp avocado oil

¼ cup (33 g) yellow onion, peeled, diced

1 garlic clove

½ cup (104 g) black beans, drained, rinsed

½ tsp ground cumin

¼ tsp chipotle powder (smoky hot) or smoked paprika

½ fresh lime, juiced

1 tbsp (3 g) fresh cilantro, chopped

4 baked eggs (see Basic Baked Eggs recipe, page 71) (smoky mild)

½ cup (57 g) reduced-fat shredded Monterey Jack-cheddar cheese blend

½ avocado

2 tbsp (30 g) plain fat-free Greek yogurt

½ cup (130 g) all-natural salsa

Heat oil in a small nonstick skillet over medium heat. Add onions and garlic and stir frequently until just translucent, about 3 minutes.

Add the black beans, cumin, chipotle powder or smoked paprika, and stir to coat.

Add lime juice and fresh cilantro and stir to combine.

Divide the beans evenly between 2 plates. Top each plate with 2 warmed baked eggs, ¼ cup (28 g) shredded cheese, ¼ avocado, 1 tablespoon (15 g) Greek yogurt and ¼ cup (65 g) salsa.

NUTRITION (PER SERVING)

Calories 280, Total Fat 11 g, Saturated Fat 3 g, Trans Fat 0 g, Cholesterol 10 mg, Sodium 290 mg, Total Carbohydrate 25 g, Dietary Fiber 9 g, Sugars 4 g, Protein 23 g, Vitamin A 10%, Vitamin C 15%, Calcium 15%, Iron 10%

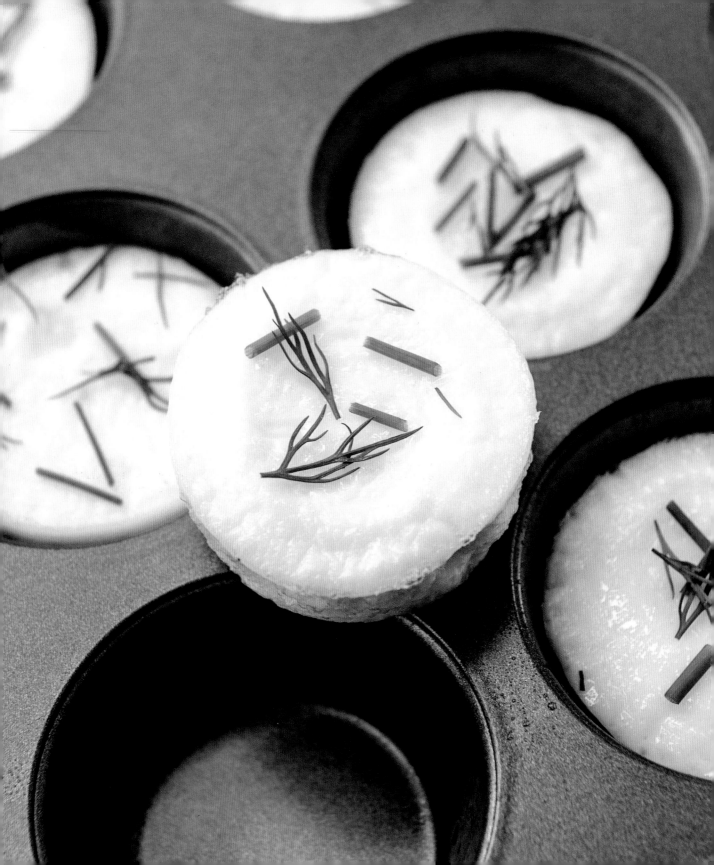

BASIC BAKED EGGS

So easy, you won't believe you've waited this long to make them! Fit them into your favorite Man Diet recipes, or partner them with fresh fruit for a simple snack.

YIELD: 6 BAKED EGGS | SERVINGS: 3 | SERVING SIZE: 2 BAKED EGGS

As needed avocado oil or spray

12 large egg whites (or 1 ½ cups [355 ml] egg whites)

Dash sea salt (optional)

Dash ground black pepper (optional)

Arrange the rack in the middle of the oven. Preheat the oven to 350°F (180°C).

Lightly coat the 6 cups of a standard nonstick muffin tin with cooking spray or avocado oil.

Place 2 egg whites or ¼ cup (60 ml) egg whites into each muffin cup.

Place the muffin pan on the middle rack. Bake for 10–15 minutes, rotating every 5 minutes to ensure even cooking.

Bake until the whites are just set. Remove from the oven and sprinkle with sea salt and black pepper if desired.

While the eggs are resting, use a plastic knife or spatula to free them from the edge of the pan. If not you're not eating immediately, allow the eggs to cool completely before storing, covered, in the refrigerator for future use.

NUTRITION (PER SERVING)
Calories 60, Total Fat 0 g, Saturated Fat 0 g, Trans Fat 0 g, Cholesterol 0 mg, Sodium 200 mg, Total Carbohydrate less than 1 g, Dietary Fiber 0 g, Sugars less than 1 g, Protein 13 g, Vitamin A 0%, Vitamin C 0%, Calcium 0%, Iron 0%

TIPS

For flavored baked eggs, try adding combinations like the following to the uncooked whites:

– Fresh tomato, fresh basil and reduced-fat shredded mozzarella cheese.

– Kalamata olives, chopped spinach, roasted red pepper, fresh mint and reduced-fat feta cheese.

– Sautéed onions, bell peppers, brown button mushrooms, fresh thyme and cheddar cheese.

FAST TRACK FRITTATA

Quick-to-make and super nutritious, this balanced option will put you on the fast track to a sustainable, high-energy day in no time. Vary your veggies, cheeses and herbs according to your preference and the season.

YIELD: 1 FRITTATA | SERVINGS: 1 | SERVING SIZE: 1 FRITTATA

- -

1 whole egg

2 egg whites

2 tbsp (5 g) fresh basil leaves, chopped

Dash sea salt

Dash ground black pepper

1 tsp avocado oil

¼ cup (33 g) yellow onion, peeled, thinly sliced

½ cup (35 g) brown button mushrooms, thinly sliced

½ cup (55 g) zucchini, thinly sliced

1 garlic clove, peeled, minced

2 tbsp (10 g) reduced-fat shredded mozzarella cheese

In a small bowl, whisk together the whole egg, egg whites, basil, salt and pepper. Set aside until needed.

In a small nonstick skillet or cast iron skillet, heat the oil over medium heat.

Add the onion and mushrooms and cook until just tender and slightly browned, about 3 minutes, stirring frequently.

Add the zucchini and garlic and cook just until tender, about 2 minutes, stirring frequently.

Spread the vegetables evenly with a spatula over the bottom of the skillet. Pour the eggs over the vegetables and cook until the bottom of the frittata has set, about 2 minutes.

Using a spatula, loosen the bottom of the pancake. Peel back one side, and tilt the pan so that the remaining uncooked egg slides to the open surface area. Using a second spatula, gently flip the frittata.

Sprinkle the cheese over the top. Cover and allow it to cook for another minute until the cheese is melted and the underside of the frittata has set.

Slide the frittata out and eat, or allow it to cool and store, covered, in the refrigerator until ready to use.

- -

NUTRITION (PER SERVING)

Calories 210, Total Fat 12 g, Saturated Fat 4 g, Trans Fat 0 g, Cholesterol 190 mg, Sodium 220 mg, Total Carbohydrate 10 g, Dietary Fiber 2 g, Sugars 5 g, Protein 16 g, Vitamin A 15%, Vitamin C 25%, Calcium 15%, Iron 8%

- -

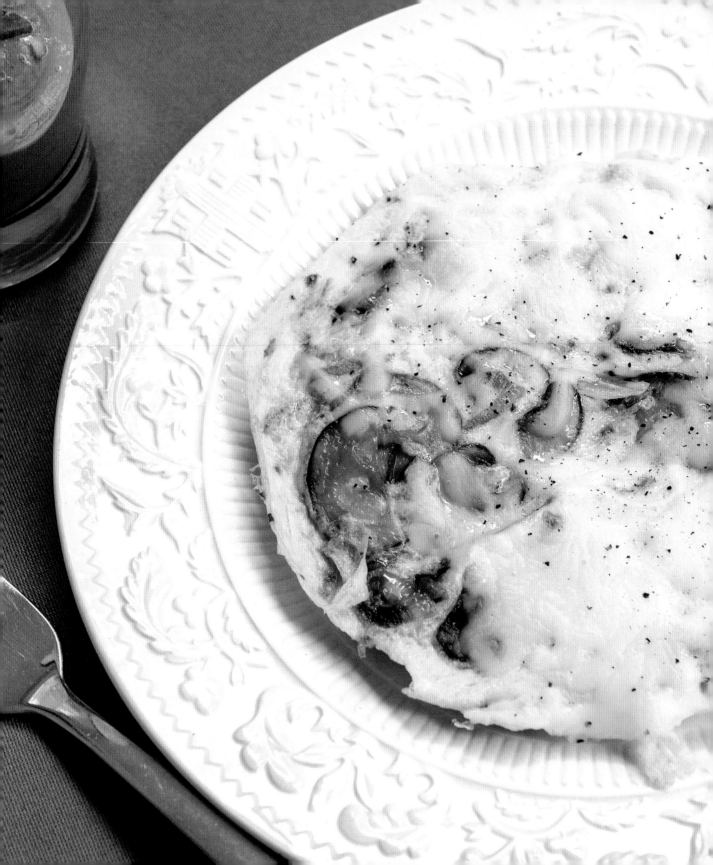

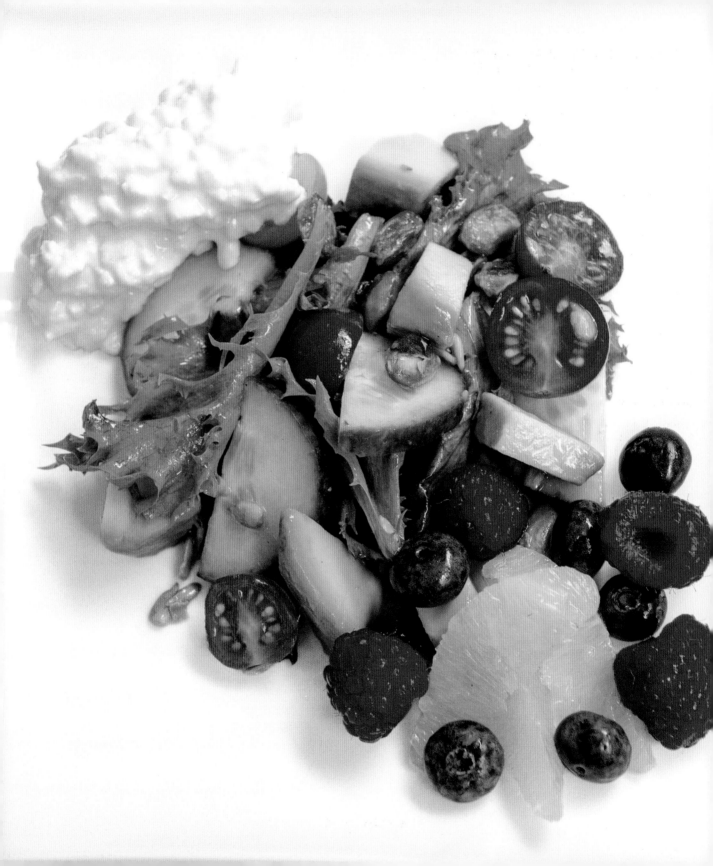

FRESH START SALAD

Light and refreshing, yet satisfying and delicious. A great way to start off any new day!

YIELD: 1 | SERVINGS: 1 | SERVING SIZE: 1 SERVING

½ tsp extra virgin olive oil

1 tsp fresh lemon juice or vinegar of choice

Dash sea salt

Dash ground black pepper

2 cups (200 g) seasonal mixed greens

3 cherry tomatoes, halved

¼ cup (26 g) cucumber, peel on, sliced

¼ avocado, diced

1 tsp nuts and seeds of choice, roasted, unsalted

¾ cup (170 g) reduced-fat cottage cheese or ricotta cheese

⅓ cup (55 g) fresh-cut mixed fruit (oranges, grapefruit, berries)

In a medium bowl, whisk together the olive oil, lemon juice or vinegar, salt and black pepper.

Add the mixed greens, tomatoes, cucumber, avocado, nuts and seeds. Toss to coat.

Place the tossed salad on a plate. Set the cottage cheese or ricotta cheese next to the salad on one side. Set the fruit salad next to the greens salad on the other side.

NUTRITION (PER SERVING)
Calories 260, Total Fat 11 g, Saturated Fat 2.5 g, Trans Fat 0 g, Cholesterol 5 mg, Sodium 40 mg, Total Carbohydrate 19 g, Dietary Fiber 5 g, Sugars 12 g, Protein 24 g, Vitamin A 100%, Vitamin C 70%, Calcium 15%, Iron 8%

GET UP & GO GRANOLA (HOMEMADE CEREAL)

Whether you pair it with milk, throw it on your yogurt, or just grab a handful on the go, this crispy, crunchy super-versatile Man Diet mix, will get you up and out and on your way toward a great day!

YIELD: 6 CUPS (174 G) | SERVINGS: 14 | SERVING SIZE: ½ CUP (15 G)

- - - - - - - - - - - - - - - - - - -

1 cup (80 g) old-fashioned rolled oats

1 ½ cups (60 g) All-Bran Buds
(I prefer Kellogg's)

1 ½ cups (60 g) SmartBran
(I prefer Nature's Path)

1 cup (137 g) nuts, dry roasted, unsalted
(pistachios, walnuts, cashews, almonds, peanuts)

1 cup (150 g) seeds, dry roasted, unsalted (sunflower, hemp, chia, sesame, flax)

¼ cup (59 ml) extra virgin olive or avocado oil

¼ cup (59 ml) 100% pure honey or 100% pure maple syrup

2 tbsp (10 g) psyllium husks
(I prefer Swanson)

1 tsp ground cinnamon

Preheat the oven to 300°F (150°C). In a large bowl, mix together all the ingredients until well combined.

Spread the granola out evenly on a rimmed baking sheet.

Bake for approximately 45 minutes, stirring every 10 minutes, until the granola is toasted.

Remove from the oven and allow it to cool completely.

Store the cooled granola in an airtight, covered container until ready to use.

- - - - - - - - - - - - - - - - - - -

NUTRITION (PER SERVING)
Calories 230, Total Fat 14 g, Saturated Fat 1.5 g, Trans Fat 0 g, Cholesterol 0 mg, Sodium 95 mg, Total Carbohydrate 26 g, Dietary Fiber 10 g, Sugars 9 g, Protein 6 g, Vitamin A 4%, Vitamin C 4%, Calcium 4%, Iron 15%

- - - - - - - - - - - - - - - - - - -

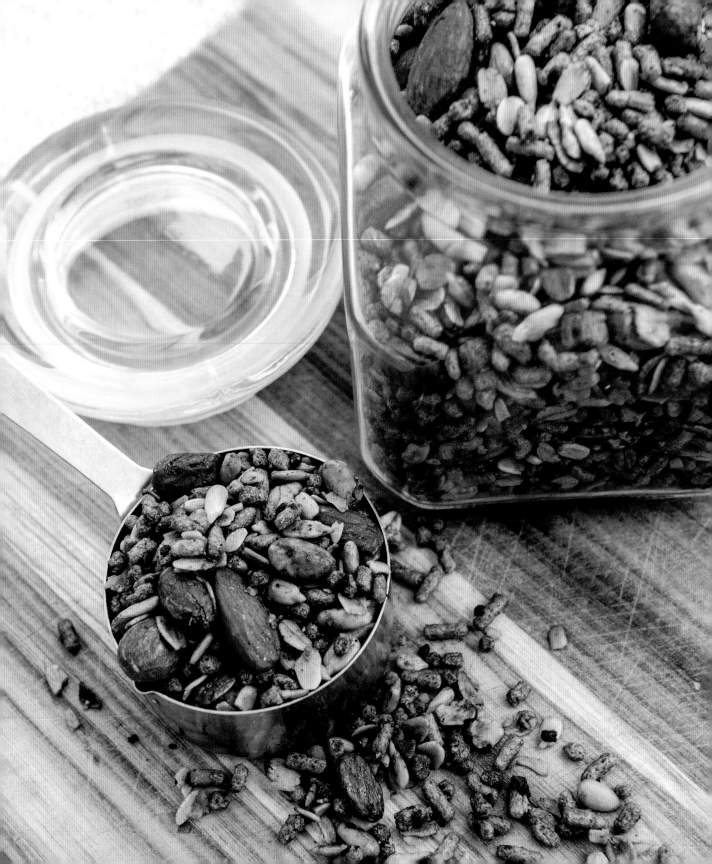

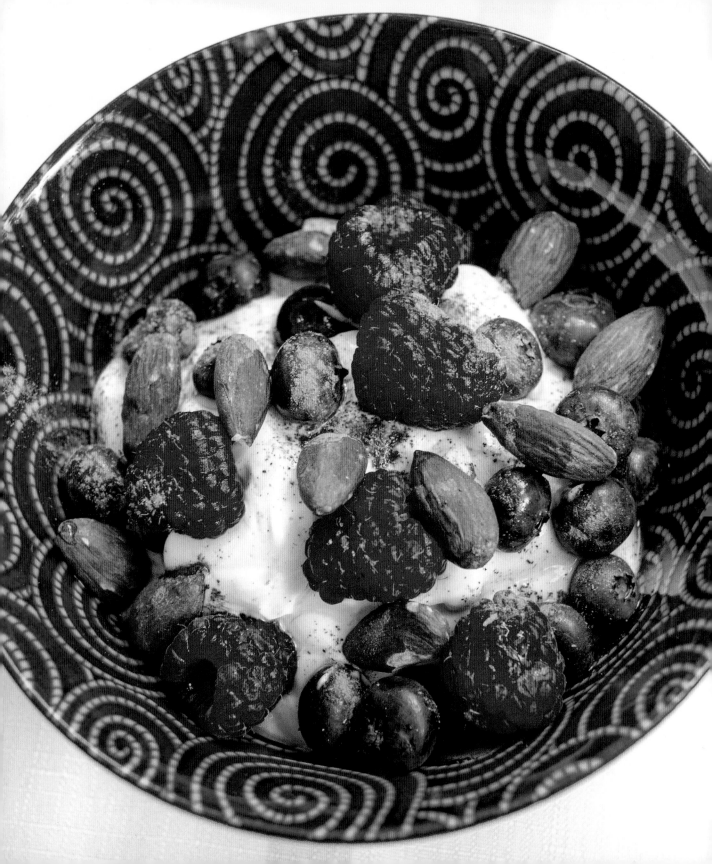

RED, WHITE AND BLUEBERRY YOGI BOWL

Even breakfast can be patriotic! Antioxidant-rich berries, crunchy almonds and cooling yogurt make this one a perfect fit for the warmer seasons. So delicious and easy, it definitely deserves a salute!

YIELD: 1 BOWL | SERVINGS: 1 | SERVING SIZE: 1 BOWL

1 cup (245 g) plain fat-free Greek yogurt

2 tbsp (21 g) almonds, roasted

¼ cup (37 g) blueberries

¼ cup (31 g) raspberries

1 tsp pure vanilla extract

½ tsp ground cinnamon

Place yogurt in a small bowl or travel container.

Top with almonds, blueberries, raspberries, vanilla extract and cinnamon.

Cover and refrigerate until ready to use.

NUTRITION (PER SERVING)
Calories 250, Total Fat 10 g, Saturated Fat 1 g, Trans Fat 0 g, Cholesterol 10 mg, Sodium 65 mg, Total Carbohydrate 20 g, Dietary Fiber 5 g, Sugars 12 g, Protein 22 g, Vitamin A 0%, Vitamin C 20%, Calcium 25%, Iron 6%

SALMON "STEAK" & EGGS WITH ASPARAGUS AND LEMON-DILL YOGURT SAUCE

Omega 3-rich salmon stars in this skillet sensation. A silky, lemony sauce and tender crisp veggies are the perfect accompaniment in this healthy take on an original classic.

YIELD: 2 | SERVINGS: 2 | SERVING SIZE: 3 OUNCES (86 G) COOKED SALMON + 2 TABLESPOONS (30 ML) SAUCE + 6 ASPARAGUS SPEARS

- -

½ cup (120 g) plain fat-free Greek yogurt

2 tsp (10 ml) extra virgin olive oil

1 tbsp (15 ml) lemon juice

½ tsp lemon zest

1 tsp fresh dill weed, chopped

¼ tsp ground black pepper

¼ tsp cayenne pepper or hot sauce

¼ tsp sea salt (optional)

2 (4-oz [115-g]) salmon fillets

12 asparagus spears, trimmed of woody ends

2 Basic Baked Eggs (page 71)

In a small bowl, whisk together the yogurt, olive oil, lemon juice, lemon zest, dill weed, black pepper, cayenne pepper or hot sauce and salt (optional), and set aside until needed.

Heat a medium nonstick skillet over medium-high heat. Add the salmon and allow it to cook covered for 3 minutes.

Gently shake the skillet to see if the salmon steaks have released from the pan. If loose, use a metal spatula to carefully flip them over.

Add the asparagus and the precooked baked eggs to the pan and cover. Cook another 3 minutes or until the salmon is cooked to desired doneness.

Remove the skillet from the heat. Divide the asparagus evenly between the two plates. Place one piece of salmon on the asparagus. Top each salmon piece with ¼ cup (61 g) yogurt sauce.

Eat or allow it to cool completely before covering and storing in the refrigerator until needed.

- -

NUTRITION (PER SERVING)
Calories 260, Total Fat 12 g, Saturated Fat 2 g, Trans Fat 0 g, Cholesterol 60 mg, Sodium 160 mg, Total Carbohydrate 6 g, Dietary Fiber 2 g, Sugars 3 g, Protein 33 g, Vitamin A 15%, Vitamin C 15%, Calcium 6%, Iron 15%

- -

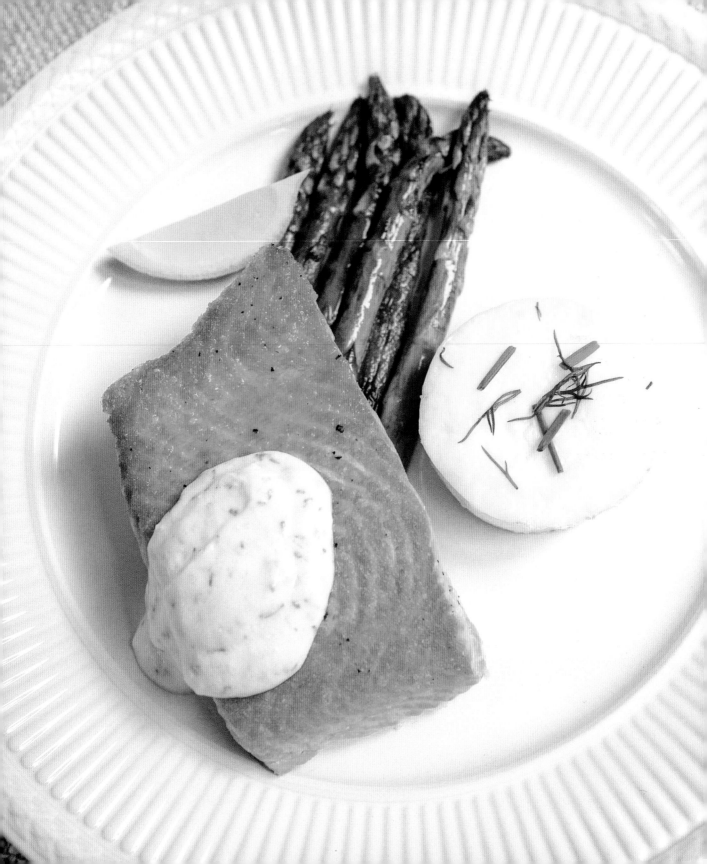

ENTRÉES

No time to prep and prepare elaborate dinners? No problem! These high-speed healthy meals will minimize your kitchen time, and free you up for fun! Make extra, and your next-day lunch is covered!

BRAISED LOW-COUNTRY PORK CHOPS

Tender chops in a rich, brothy sauce are not easy to resist. Thank goodness you don't have to here. Moist-heat cooking makes all the difference with this succulent dish!

YIELD: 4 | SERVINGS: 4 | SERVING SIZE: 3 OUNCES (85 G) PORK + ¾ CUP (170 G) VEGETABLES

½ tsp ground black pepper

½ tsp dry thyme leaves

½ tsp paprika

½ tsp garlic powder

½ tsp onion powder

4 (4-oz [113-g]) boneless pork loin chops, trimmed of visible fat

2 tsp (10 ml) avocado oil, divided

4 cups (237 g) brown button mushrooms, quartered

2 cups (300 g) yellow onion, peeled, chopped medium

2 cups (202 g) celery, chopped medium

3 garlic cloves, peeled, minced

3 cups (713 ml) fat-free, low-sodium chicken stock

1 dry bay leaf

2 tbsp (30 g) coarse-ground mustard

Combine the black pepper, thyme, paprika, garlic powder and onion powder in a small cup, mixing to combine.

Rub the spice mixture on both sides of the pork chops until coated. Wash your hands with soap and water to clean.

In a large heavy-bottomed skillet, heat 1 teaspoon avocado oil over medium-high heat. Cook the pork for 2 minutes on each side or until browned. (The pork is not completely cooked at this point.) Transfer the pork chops to a separate plate until ready.

In the same skillet, still over medium-high heat, heat the remaining avocado oil. Add the mushrooms, onion, celery and garlic and cook for 3 minutes or until vegetables are just beginning to soften, stirring occasionally.

Add the broth, bay leaf and mustard, and stir to combine. Add the pork chops back to the skillet.

Cover, reduce the heat and simmer for about 20 minutes or until the pork is cooked through and no pink is remaining. Remove the skillet from the heat, and transfer the pork chops to a separate clean plate. Cover to keep warm.

Increase the heat to high and return the skillet to the stovetop. Cook for 5 minutes or until the volume is reduced to 3 cups (713 ml) liquid and vegetables.

Serve the cooked pork chops with the vegetable mixture spooned over the top. If not eating immediately, allow it to cool completely before storing it, tightly covered, in the refrigerator until ready to use.

NUTRITION (PER SERVING)
Calories 270, Total Fat 11 g, Saturated Fat 3.5 g, Trans Fat 0 g, Cholesterol 60 mg, Sodium 320 mg, Total Carbohydrate 12 g, Dietary Fiber 3 g, Sugars 5 g, Protein 29 g, Vitamin A 8%, Vitamin C 10%, Calcium 6%, Iron 10%

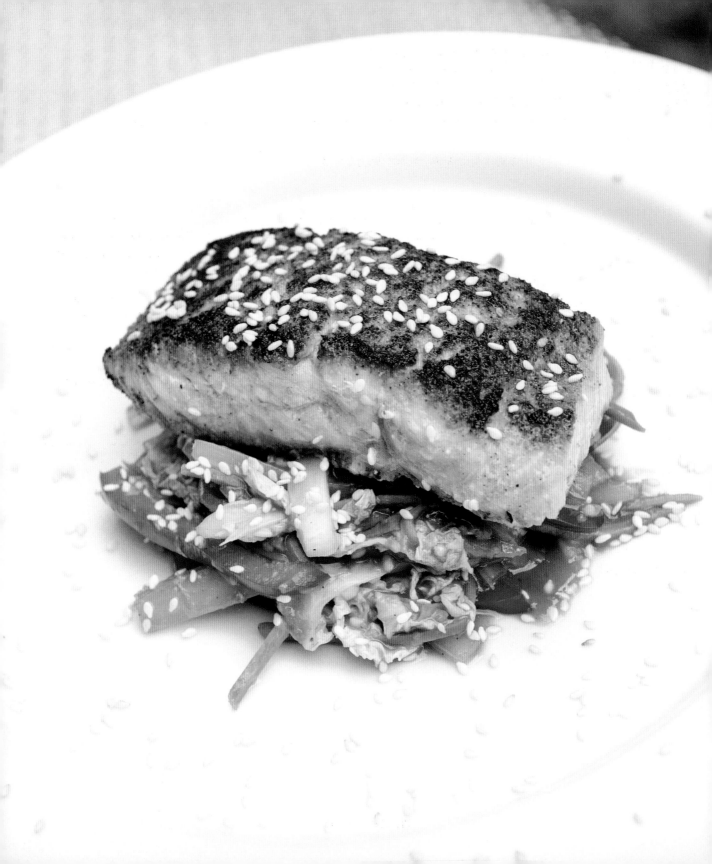

FIVE-SPICE SEARED SALMON WITH MU SHU VEGETABLES

Tender crisp vegetables provide a satisfying foundation for fragrant seared salmon. Five incredible spices yield one out-of-this-world dish!

YIELD: 4 | SERVINGS: 4 | SERVING SIZE: 3 OUNCES (86 G) SALMON + 1 CUP (128 G) VEGETABLES

4 (4-oz [115-g]) wild salmon fillet

1 tsp Chinese five-spice powder

2 tsp (10 ml) avocado oil

2 garlic cloves, peeled, minced

1 tsp fresh ginger, minced

1 cup (101 g) celery, cut into matchsticks

1 cup (122 g) carrots, peeled, cut into matchsticks

1 cup (87 g) fennel bulb, cut into matchsticks

1 cup (70 g) napa cabbage, cut into strips

1 cup (175 g) red bell peppers, seeded, cut into matchsticks

2 tbsp (30 ml) reduced-sodium soy sauce

1 tbsp (15 ml) hoisin sauce

1 cup (50 g) scallions, green part only

1 tbsp (8 g) toasted sesame seeds

Dust each salmon fillet with five-spice powder to coat. Heat a large nonstick skillet over medium-high heat. Place each salmon fillet in the pan and allow it to cook for 4 minutes. Turn the salmon with a spatula and cook another 4 minutes or until desired doneness. Remove the salmon to a side plate until needed.

With the skillet still on medium high, add the avocado oil. Add the garlic, ginger, celery, carrots, fennel bulb, cabbage and red pepper. Cook, stirring vegetables regularly until the vegetables are just tender crisp, about 4 minutes.

Add the soy sauce, hoisin and scallions to the vegetables and stir to coat.

Serve the vegetables with the salmon on top. Sprinkle the sesame seeds evenly over the top of each dish.

NUTRITION (PER SERVING)

Calories 250, Total Fat 11 g, Saturated Fat 1.5 g, Trans Fat 0 g, Cholesterol 60 mg, Sodium 450 mg, Total Carbohydrate 13 g, Dietary Fiber 4 g, Sugars 5 g, Protein 25 g, Vitamin A 160%, Vitamin C 110%, Calcium 8%, Iron 10%

ALLSPICE-RUBBED PORK TENDERLOIN WITH BRAISED RED CABBAGE AND GRAIN MUSTARD

A perfect comfort dish for a cool evening. Savory allspice works great with chicken breast too!

YIELD: 4 | SERVINGS: 4 | SERVING SIZE: 3 OUNCES (85 G) PORK + 1 CUP (70 G) CABBAGE

- -

1 tbsp (7 g) ground allspice

½ tsp sea salt (optional)

1 tsp ground black pepper

1 lb (454 g) pork tenderloin, trimmed of all visible fat

3 tsp (15 ml) avocado oil

1 ½ cups (195 g) yellow onion, peeled, thinly sliced

4 cups (280 g) red cabbage, thinly sliced

¼ cup (59 ml) red wine vinegar

1 tbsp (15 ml) 100% pure honey

1 tsp ground cinnamon

1 cup (237 ml) dry red wine

1 cup (238 ml) fat-free, low-sodium chicken stock

¼ cup (59 ml) grain mustard

Combine the allspice, ¼ teaspoon sea salt and ½ teaspoon black pepper in a small cup. On a large plate, rub the spice mix over the pork tenderloin to coat thoroughly. Allow it to stand for 30 minutes.

In a large skillet heat 2 teaspoons (10 ml) oil over medium heat. Cook the onion for 5 minutes or just until soft, stirring frequently.

Stir in the cabbage, vinegar, honey, cinnamon, red wine and chicken stock. Bring to a simmer and cook covered for 15 minutes or until the cabbage is softened. Remove the cover and continue to cook over medium heat until most of the liquid is gone, about 5 minutes, stirring occasionally. Remove from the heat and cover to keep warm.

In a separate heavy-bottomed skillet, heat the remainder of the oil, swirling to coat the pan, over medium-high heat. Add the pork tenderloin and cook for about 20 minutes, turning every 5 minutes or until the internal temperature reads 145°F (63°C) on an instant-read thermometer. Remove from the heat and allow it to rest for 5 minutes before slicing.

Slice the cooked pork tenderloin crosswise into pieces. Serve atop the braised cabbage with 1 tablespoon (15 ml) grain mustard for garnish.

- -

NUTRITION (PER SERVING)
Calories 290, Total Fat 8 g, Saturated Fat 1.5 g, Trans Fat 0 g, Cholesterol 60 mg, Sodium 360 mg, Total Carbohydrate 17 g, Dietary Fiber 3 g, Sugars 9 g, Protein 25 g, Vitamin A 20%, Vitamin C 80%, Calcium 8%, Iron 10%

- -

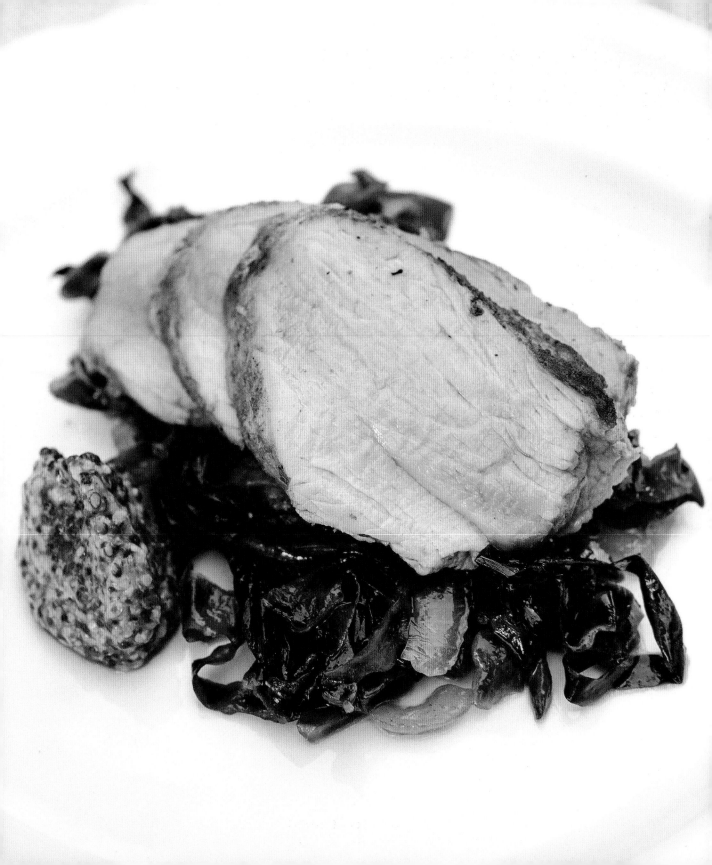

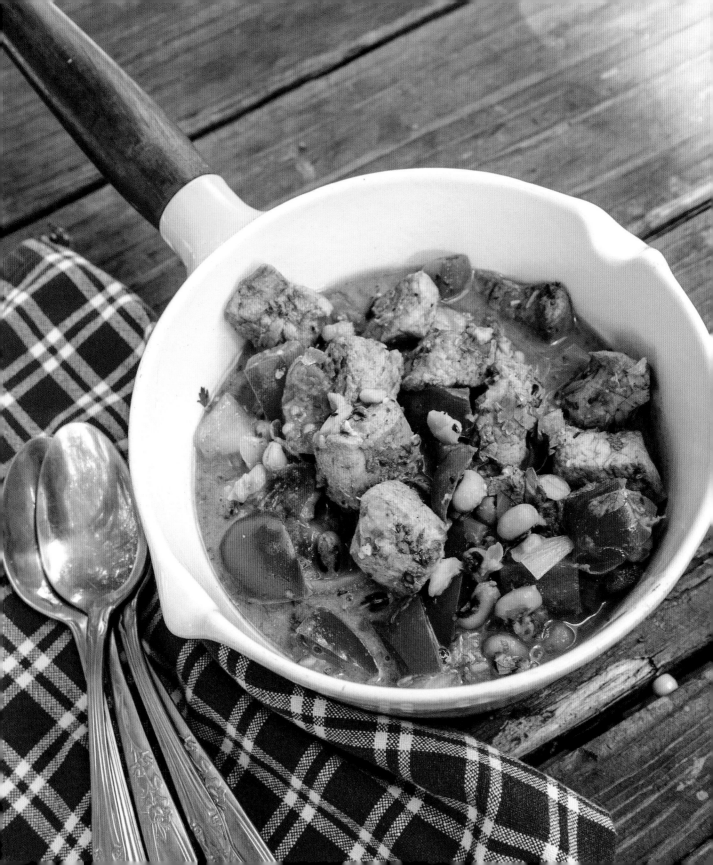

ANCHO PORK AND PINTO BEAN STEW

This fireside classic comes out of the campsite and into your kitchen. Repurpose any leftovers for a healthy weekend breakfast by topping with baked eggs.

YIELD: 4 CUPS (1 L) | **SERVINGS: 4** | **SERVING SIZE: 1 CUP (237 ML)**

---

1 lb (454 g) pork tenderloin, trimmed of visible fat, cut into ½-inch (1.3-cm) square pieces

1 ½ tbsp (11 g) ground ancho chili powder

1 tsp dried oregano leaves

1 tsp smoked paprika

½ tsp ground cumin

½ tsp black pepper

¼ tsp sea salt (optional)

1 tbsp (15 ml) avocado oil, divided

1 ½ cups (195 g) yellow onion, peeled, chopped medium

3 garlic cloves, peeled, minced

¾ cup (130 g) green bell pepper, seeded, chopped medium

¾ cup (130 g) red bell pepper, seeded, chopped medium

2 cups (475 ml) fat-free, low-sodium chicken stock

2 cups (360 g) red ripe tomatoes, chopped medium

2 tsp (10 ml) Dijon mustard

1 tsp apple cider vinegar

1 cup (201 g) pinto beans, drained, rinsed

2 tbsp (6 g) fresh cilantro

Combine pork tenderloin, chili powder, oregano, paprika, cumin, black pepper and salt (optional) in a medium bowl. Toss to coat thoroughly

Heat half the oil in a large heavy-bottomed stockpot over medium-high heat. Add the pork mixture and cook 5 minutes or until browned, stirring occasionally. Remove the pork from the pan with a slotted spoon and set aside.

Add the remainder of the oil to the pan. Add the onion, garlic and bell peppers and sauté for 5 minutes or until just tender, stirring occasionally.

Return the pork to the pan. Add the stock, tomatoes, mustard, vinegar and beans. Bring to a boil. Partially cover, reduce heat and simmer for 20 minutes.

Remove from the heat and stir in the fresh cilantro.

Serve immediately or allow it to cool fully before storing it, tightly covered, in the refrigerator until ready to use.

NUTRITION (PER SERVING)
Calories 270, Total Fat 6 g, Saturated Fat 1.5 g, Trans Fat 0 g, Cholesterol 60 mg, Sodium 350 mg, Total Carbohydrate 24 g, Dietary Fiber 8 g, Sugars 6 g, Protein 29 g, Vitamin A 60%, Vitamin C 110%, Calcium 8%, Iron 20%

BISON HANGER STEAK WITH CHIMICHURRI AND GRILLED CARROTS

Tender, quick-cooking hanger gets a flavor boost from pungent, herbaceous chimichurri sauce. The carrots cook right alongside for convenience.

YIELD: 4 | SERVINGS: 4 | SERVING SIZE: 1 STEAK + 1 CUP (122 G) CARROTS + ¼ CUP (68 G) CHIMICHURRI SAUCE | YIELD: ABOUT 2 CUPS (546 G)

SAUCE

3 garlic cloves, peeled, minced

1 serrano chili, (seeded for less heat), minced

1 ¼ cups (50 g) flat-leaf parsley leaves, chopped

½ cup (25 g) fresh cilantro leaves, chopped

3 tbsp (8 g) fresh oregano leaves, chopped

½ cup (120 ml) extra virgin olive oil

2 tbsp (30 ml) apple cider vinegar

½ tsp sea salt (optional)

½ tsp ground black pepper

¼ cup (59 ml) fat-free, low-sodium chicken stock

1 lb (454 g) bison hanger tender steak, trimmed of all visible fat, cut into 4 steaks

1 tsp ground black pepper

4 large carrots, peeled, cut lengthwise into ½-inch (1-cm) thick strips

1 tsp avocado oil

In a medium bowl combine the garlic, chili, parsley, cilantro and oregano. Add the oil, vinegar, ½ teaspoon each of salt (optional) and black pepper, and chicken stock, stirring to combine. Set aside the chimichurri sauce until needed.

Heat a grill to medium high. Season both sides of steaks with 1 teaspoon black pepper. Toss carrots in a medium bowl with avocado oil. Place steaks and carrots on the grill and cook until desired doneness. Cook 3–4 minutes each side for medium-rare (suggested doneness). Carrots will be just fork tender. Remove steaks and carrots from the grill.

Divide the steak and carrots between 4 plates. Top with chimichurri sauce and serve. If not serving immediately, allow it to cool completely before tightly covering and storing in the refrigerator.

NUTRITION (PER SERVING)

Calories 290, Total Fat 16 g, Saturated Fat 2.5 g, Trans Fat 0 g, Cholesterol 70 mg, Sodium 240 mg, Total Carbohydrate 9 g, Dietary Fiber 3 g, Sugars 4 g, Protein 29 g, Vitamin A 260%, Vitamin C 30%, Calcium 6%, Iron 25%

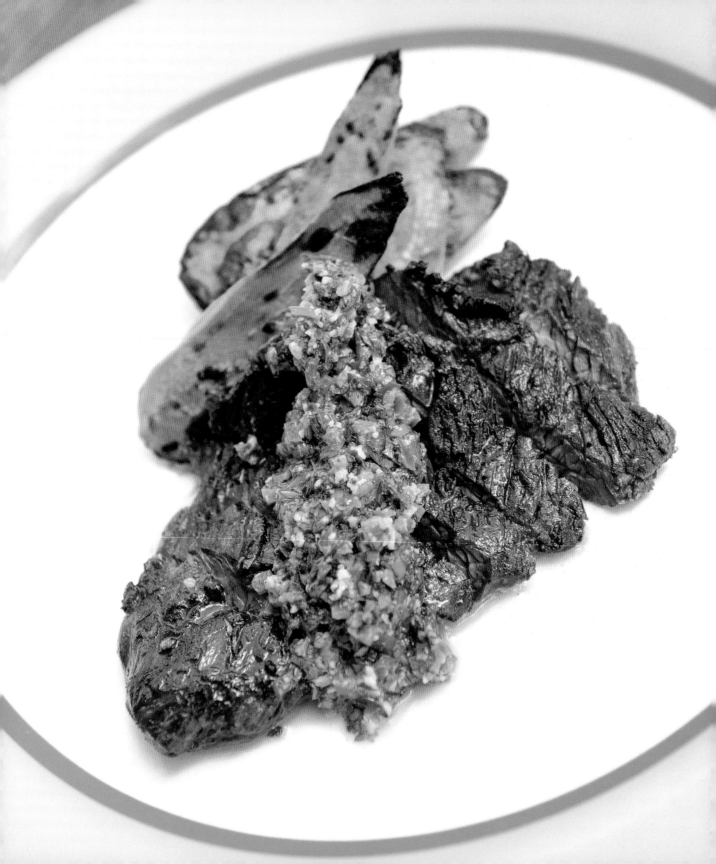

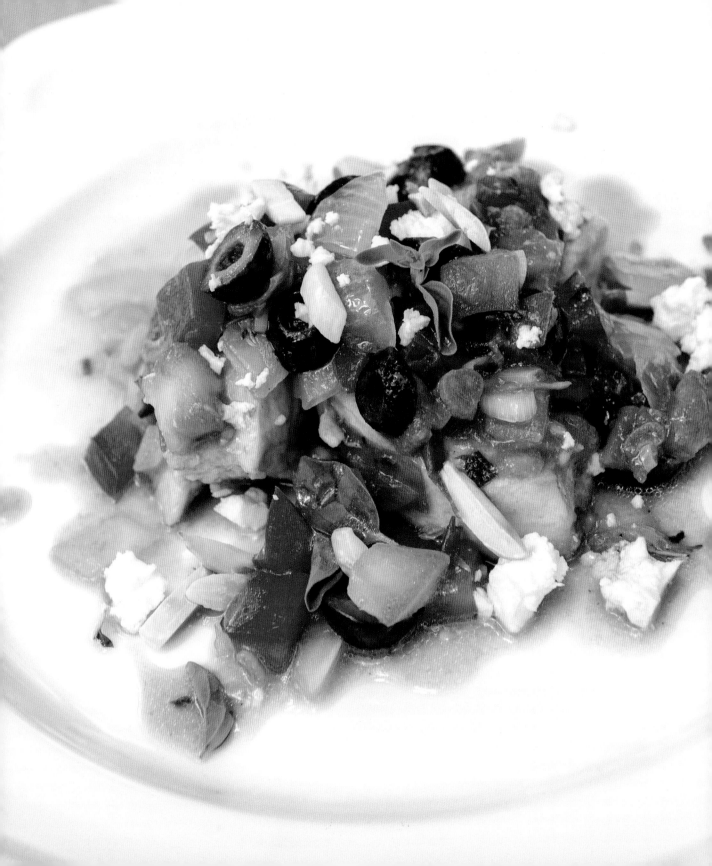

CHICKEN OREGANATA

The flavors of the Mediterranean shine through in this dish. Perfect with fresh fish, too!

YIELD: 8 CUPS (1 L) | SERVINGS: 4 | SERVING SIZE: 2 CUPS (300 G) + 1 TABLESPOON (9 G) FETA

2 tsp (10 ml) avocado oil

1 lb (454 g) chicken breast, boneless, skinless, trimmed of visible fat, cut into 2-inch (5-cm) cubes

1 cup (150 g) yellow onion, peeled, chopped medium

1 cup (175 g) red bell pepper, seeded, chopped medium

4 garlic cloves, peeled, minced

½ cup (25 g) scallion, green part only, chopped small

1 cup (180 g) red ripe tomatoes, chopped medium

¼ tsp crushed red chili flakes

1 tbsp (3 g) fresh oregano leaves, chopped

2 tbsp (30 ml) lemon juice

½ cup (119 ml) dry white wine

1 cup (238 ml) fat-free, low-sodium chicken stock

¼ cup (45 g) sliced black olives, drained, rinsed

1 tbsp (15 ml) extra virgin olive oil

½ tsp ground black pepper

¼ cup (30 g) roasted slivered almonds

¼ cup (38 g) reduced-fat feta cheese

Heat the avocado oil over medium-high heat in a large nonstick skillet. Add the chicken and cook until no pink remains in the center, stirring regularly for about 8 minutes.

Add the onion, bell peppers, garlic and scallion, and cook 4 minutes, stirring regularly until the onions are just tender crisp.

Add the tomatoes, crushed chili flakes and oregano leaves, and stir to combine, cooking another 2 minutes.

Add the lemon juice, dry white wine and chicken stock, and simmer until the liquid is reduced by half, about 4 minutes.

Fold in the black olives, olive oil, black pepper and almonds, and cook for another 2 minutes. The chicken should be fully cooked and registering 165°F (74°C) on an instant-read thermometer.

Divide between 4 separate dishes and garnish each with 1 tablespoon (9 g) feta cheese.

NUTRITION (PER SERVING)
Calories 330, Total Fat 15 g, Saturated Fat 3 g, Trans Fat 0 g, Cholesterol 90 mg, Sodium 280 mg, Total Carbohydrate 12 g, Dietary Fiber 4 g, Sugars 5 g, Protein 32 g, Vitamin A 35%, Vitamin C 100%, Calcium 8%, Iron 10%

CHICKEN TIKKA MASALA WITH ROASTED CAULIFLOWER

This simplified version of the Indian classic is easy to get marinating the night before or in the morning, so it's full-flavored and ready to roll when you're ready to cook! Nutty roasted cauliflower makes the perfect accompaniment. Roast extra and you have the beginnings for your Curried Cauliflower Soup (page 127)!

YIELD: 4 | SERVINGS: 4 | SERVING SIZE: 3 OUNCES (85 G) CHICKEN + 1 CUP (100 G) CAULIFLOWER

- -

1 cup (225 ml) all-natural tomato sauce

1 cup (245 g) plain fat-free Greek yogurt

½ tsp fresh ginger, minced

2 tbsp (13 g) curry powder

½ tsp ground cumin

1 cup (100 g) scallions, sliced thin

¼ tsp sea salt (optional)

½ tsp ground black pepper

1 ½ lbs (680 g) chicken breast, boneless, skinless, trimmed of all visible fat

5 cups (500 g) medium cauliflower florets

2 tsp (10 ml) avocado oil

2 tbsp (30 ml) fresh lemon juice

2 tbsp (6 g) fresh cilantro leaves, chopped

In a medium bowl, combine the tomato sauce, yogurt, ginger, curry powder, cumin, scallions, salt (optional) and ground black pepper. Mix to combine. Add the chicken and turn to coat thoroughly. Marinate covered in the refrigerator for at least 1 hour.

In a medium bowl toss the cauliflower with the avocado oil to coat. Spread evenly onto a baking sheet and set aside until needed.

Preheat the oven to 375°F (190°C). Transfer the chicken from the marinade to a medium-sized ovenproof glass dish. Cover with foil. Place the chicken in the oven and bake for about 1 hour or until the chicken is fully cooked and the internal temperature of the chicken reads 165°F (74°C) with an instant-read thermometer.

Halfway through the chicken cooking time, place the cauliflower in the oven and bake until just tender.

Remove the cauliflower from the oven, transfer to a bowl and toss with the lemon juice and cilantro.

Remove the chicken from the oven.

Divide the cauliflower evenly among 4 plates and top with 1 piece of chicken. If not eating immediately, allow it to cool completely before storing it, tightly covered, in the refrigerator until it's ready to use.

- -

NUTRITION (PER SERVING)
Calories 260, Total Fat 8 g, Saturated Fat 1.5 g, Trans Fat 0 g, Cholesterol 90 mg, Sodium 310 mg, Total Carbohydrate 14 g, Dietary Fiber 4 g, Sugars 6 g, Protein 34 g, Vitamin A 10%, Vitamin C 110%, Calcium 10%, Iron 15%

- -

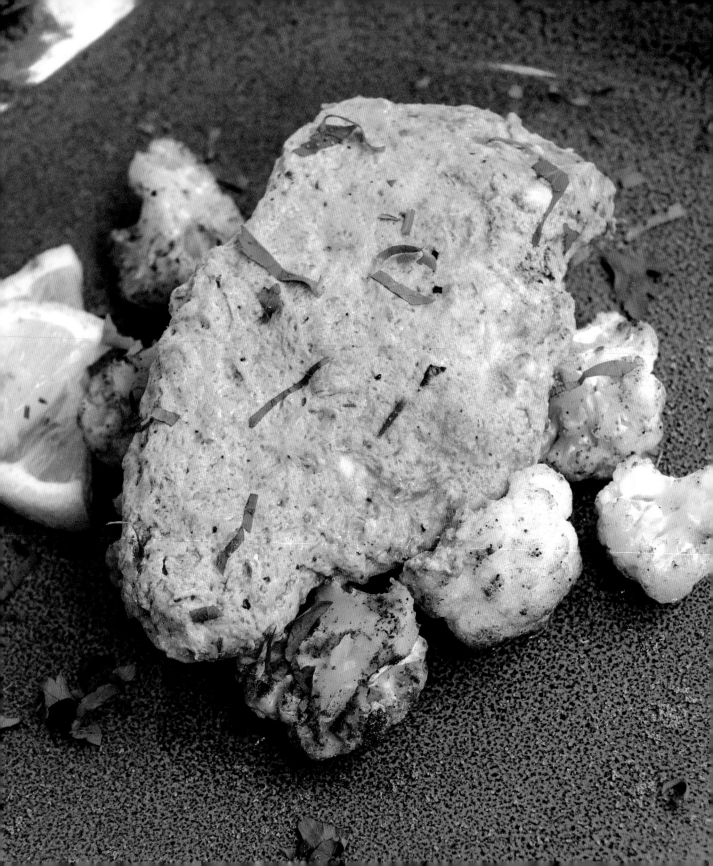

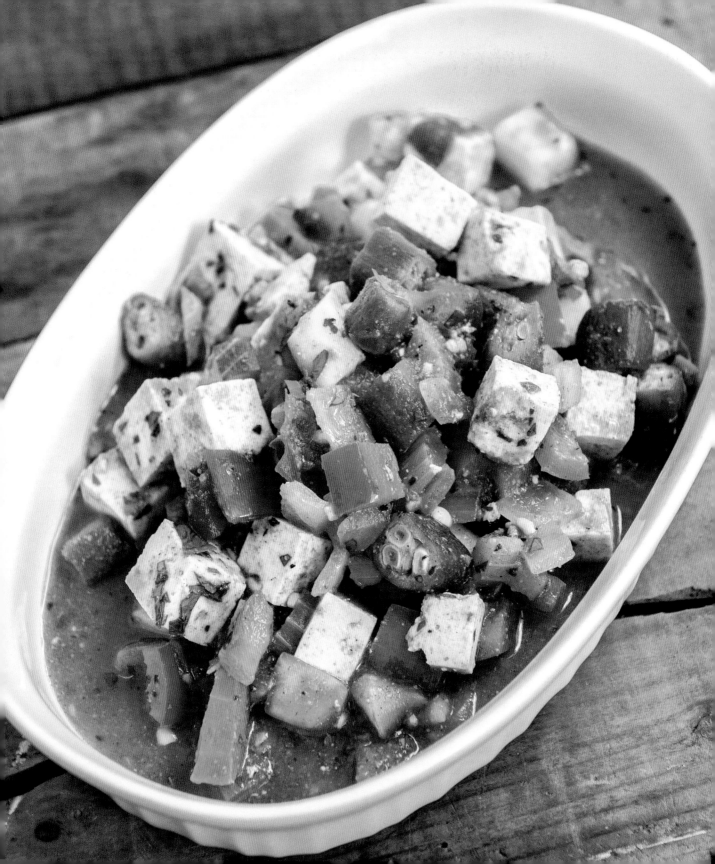

CREOLE TOFU-VEGETABLE ÉTOUFÉE

A true party in a pot! Soft tofu teams with fragrant creole flavors in this hearty, vegetable-rich dish. So delicious you'll swear it's Mardi Gras every time you make it!

YIELD 7 CUPS (1.5 L) | **SERVINGS 4** | **SERVING SIZE 1 ¾ CUPS (414 ML)**

2 tbsp (30 ml) avocado oil

1 cup (101 g) celery, chopped medium

1 cup (150 g) yellow onion, chopped medium

1 cup (128 g) carrots, peeled, chopped medium

1 cup (175 g) red bell peppers, seeded, chopped medium

1 cup (175 g) green bell peppers, seeded, chopped medium

3 garlic cloves, peeled, minced

1 ½ cups (270 g) red ripe tomatoes, chopped medium

1 cup (238 ml) fat-free, low-sodium vegetable broth

2 cups (200 g) frozen sliced okra, thawed

1 (140-oz [395-g]) package extra-firm tofu, drained, chopped medium

1 cup (110 g) zucchini

½ cup (125 ml) tomato purée

2 bay leaves

1 tsp dried thyme

1 tsp filé powder (optional)

½ tsp chili powder

½ tsp ground cumin

½ tsp onion powder

½ tsp garlic powder

½ tsp paprika

½ tsp ground black pepper

¼ tsp ground cayenne pepper

¼ tsp sea salt (optional)

In a large skillet or soup pot, heat the oil over medium-low heat. Add the celery, onion, carrot, bell peppers and garlic. Cook for 5 minutes, stirring occasionally.

Increase the heat to medium and stir in the tomatoes and broth. Cover and cook for 10 minutes, stirring occasionally.

Stir in the remaining ingredients. Bring to a simmer. Cover and simmer for 10 minutes or until the vegetables are just tender. Discard the bay leaves before serving.

NUTRITION (PER SERVING)

Calories 260, Total Fat 12 g, Saturated Fat 1.5 g, Trans Fat 0 g, Cholesterol 0 mg, Sodium 260 mg, Total Carbohydrate 28 g, Dietary Fiber 9 g, Sugars 14 g, Protein 13 g, Vitamin A 170%, Vitamin C 170%, Calcium 20%, Iron 25%

GRILLED CHICKEN ENCHILADA WITH SUMMER SQUASH AND CHILI ROJA

Grilled, moist chicken and bright summer squashes, all smothered in a rich tomato sauce with pungent cheddar, will help you forget this easy-to-assemble dish is tortilla free.

YIELD: 4 | SERVINGS: 4 | SERVING SIZE: 3 OUNCES (85 G) CHICKEN + ½ CUP (64 G) VEGETABLES + ½ CUP (118 G) SAUCE + 1 TABLESPOON (7 G) CHEESE + 1 TABLESPOON (15 G) YOGURT + ¼ AVOCADO

CHICKEN

1 tbsp (15 ml) avocado oil

1 tbsp (15 ml) fresh lime juice

2 tbsp (6 g) fresh cilantro

¼ tsp sea salt (optional)

½ tsp ground black pepper

2 garlic cloves, peeled and chopped

1 lb (454 g) chicken breast, boneless, skinless, cut into 4-oz (113-g) pieces

SQUASH

1 medium zucchini squash, cut on the bias, 1-inch (3-cm) thick slices

1 medium yellow squash, cut on the bias, 1-inch (3-cm) thick slices

2 tsp (10 ml) avocado oil

SAUCE

1 cup (225 ml) tomato sauce

1 cup (238 ml) fat-free, low-sodium chicken stock

1 tbsp (16 g) ground cumin

2 tsp (5 g) ground chipotle powder

¼ cup (28 g) reduced-fat shredded cheddar cheese

1 fresh avocado, peeled and quartered

¼ cup (61 g) plain, fat-free Greek yogurt

Combine the avocado oil, lime juice, cilantro, salt (optional), black pepper and garlic in a medium square glass dish. Add the chicken and turn to coat. Cover and marinate in the refrigerator for an hour.

Preheat the grill to medium. In a medium bowl, toss the zucchini and yellow squash with the avocado oil. Set aside until needed.

In a medium-size, heavy-bottomed saucepan, bring the tomato sauce, chicken stock, cumin and chipotle powder to a boil. Reduce the heat and simmer until the liquid is reduced by half the amount, about 4 minutes. Remove from the heat and cover to keep warm.

Place the chicken on the grill and cook for about 10 minutes, flipping after 5 minutes, until cooked through and juices run clear. The internal temperature will read 165°F (74°C) on an instant-read thermometer. Add the squash to the grill halfway through the chicken cooking time. Flip after 2 ½ minutes.

Remove the chicken and the squash from the grill. Divide the squash evenly among 4 plates. Top each plate with 1 piece of chicken, ½ cup (115 g) roja sauce, 1 tablespoon (7 g) cheddar cheese, ¼ avocado and 1 tablespoon (15 g) yogurt.

NUTRITION (PER SERVING)
Calories 320, Total Fat 18 g, Saturated Fat 3 g, Trans Fat 0 g, Cholesterol 90 mg, Sodium 340 mg, Total Carbohydrate 10 g, Dietary Fiber 4 g, Sugars 4 g, Protein 32 g, Vitamin A 20%, Vitamin C 30%, Calcium 10%, Iron 16%

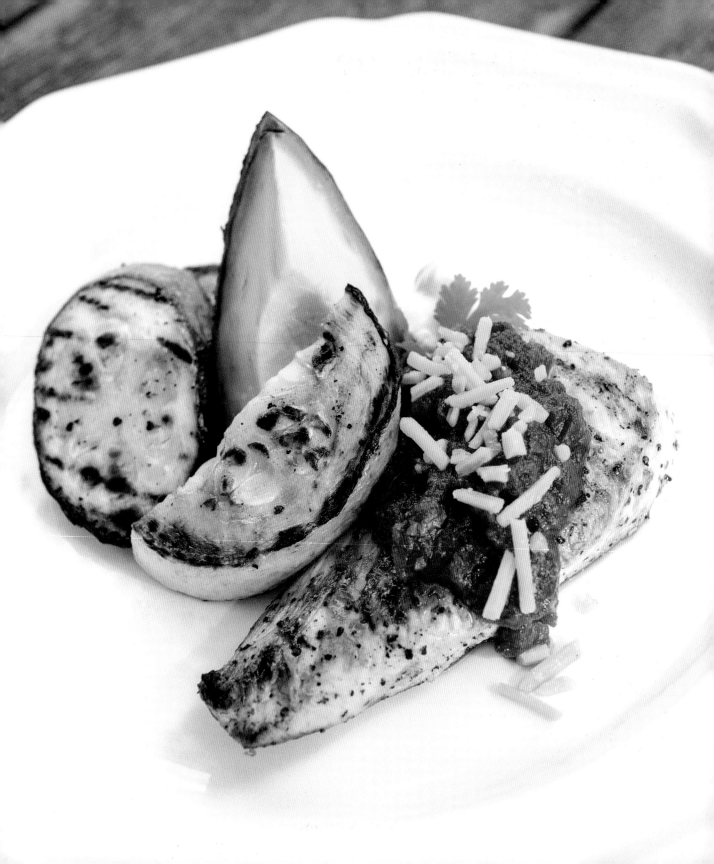

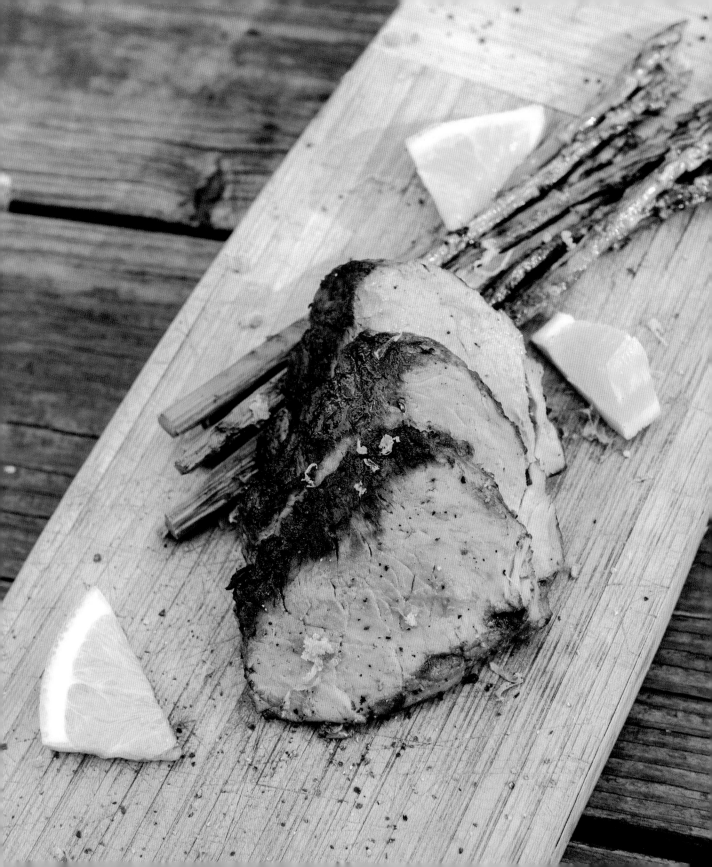

GRILLED SWEET CHILI PORK TENDERLOIN WITH ASPARAGUS

A spicy, sweet, and sour marinade transforms lean pork tenderloin into a BBQ grilled masterpiece. Savory and smoky grilled asparagus provides nice balance to the dish.

YIELD: 4 | SERVINGS: 4 | SERVING SIZE: 3 OUNCES (85 G) COOKED PORK + 8 ASPARAGUS

32 asparagus spears, trimmed of hard ends

3 tsp (15 ml) avocado oil

¼ cup (59 ml) unseasoned rice vinegar

2 tbsp (30 ml) 100% pure honey

¼ tsp salt

3 tsp (15 ml) toasted sesame oil

2 tsp (11 ml) Sriracha hot chili sauce

¼ cup (13 g) fresh cilantro leaves, chopped

1 tbsp (6 g) orange zest

2 garlic cloves

1 lb (454 g) pork tenderloin, trimmed of visible fat

Cooking spray as needed

On a plate, gently toss the asparagus with 1 ½ teaspoons (7 ml) of avocado oil to coat. Set aside.

In a large glass dish, combine the vinegar, honey, salt, sesame oil, chili sauce, 1 ½ teaspoons (7 ml) avocado oil, cilantro, orange zest and garlic. Add the pork tenderloin, turning to coat. Cover tightly and refrigerate for 2 hours, turning occasionally.

Preheat the grill to medium. Spray the grate with cooking spray. Drain the pork, discarding the marinade. Grill the pork on all sides, turning roughly every 5 minutes (the pork should pull easily away from the grill), for about 20 minutes or until the internal temperature reads 145°F (63°C) with an instant-read thermometer.

Add the asparagus to the grill during the last 5 minutes of the pork's cooking time. Turn the asparagus occasionally.

Remove the pork and asparagus from the grill, and allow to rest for 5 minutes before cutting.

Cut the pork crosswise into slices and serve atop the asparagus. If not eating immediately, allow it to cool completely before storing it, tightly covered, in the refrigerator.

NUTRITION (PER SERVING)
Calories 290, Total Fat 10 g, Saturated Fat 2 g, Trans Fat 0 g, Cholesterol 60 mg, Sodium 300 mg, Total Carbohydrate 17 g, Dietary Fiber 4 g, Sugars 12 g, Protein 26 g, Vitamin A 25%, Vitamin C 20%, Calcium 6%, Iron 30%

HOPPIN' JOE

Frozen collards and canned black-eyed peas help to keep things high-quality, but simple, in this Southern superstar. Just one pot makes for minimal cleanup too!

YIELD: 8 CUPS (2 L) | SERVINGS: 4 | SERVING SIZE: 2 CUPS (473 ML)

- -

2 tsp (10 ml) avocado oil

½ cup (75 g) onion, chopped medium

½ cup (51 g) celery, chopped medium

½ cup (90 g) red bell pepper, seeded, chopped medium

½ cup (90 g) yellow bell pepper, seeded, chopped medium

2 garlic cloves, peeled, minced

4 cups (952 ml) fat-free, low-sodium chicken broth

1 ½ cups (150 g) frozen chopped collard greens, thawed

1 cup (240 g) black-eyed peas, drained, rinsed

2 cups (360 g) red ripe tomatoes, chopped

12 oz (341 g) grilled chicken breast, chopped medium

½ tsp chili powder

½ tsp ground cumin

½ tsp onion powder

½ tsp garlic powder

½ tsp paprika

½ tsp ground black pepper

¼ tsp ground cayenne pepper (optional)

¼ tsp sea salt (optional)

In a large soup pot, heat the oil over medium-high heat. Cook the onion, celery, bell peppers and garlic for 5 minutes or until the vegetables are just tender, stirring occasionally.

Stir in the remaining ingredients and bring to a simmer. Cook for another 10 minutes.

Remove from the heat and serve or cool completely before storing, covered tightly, in the refrigerator.

- -

NUTRITION (PER SERVING)
Calories 270, Total Fat 6 g, Saturated Fat 1 g, Trans Fat 0 g, Cholesterol 90 mg, Sodium 320 mg, Total Carbohydrate 23 g, Dietary Fiber 7 g, Sugars 6 g, Protein 35 g, Vitamin A 180%, Vitamin C 160%, Calcium 15%, Iron 15%

- -

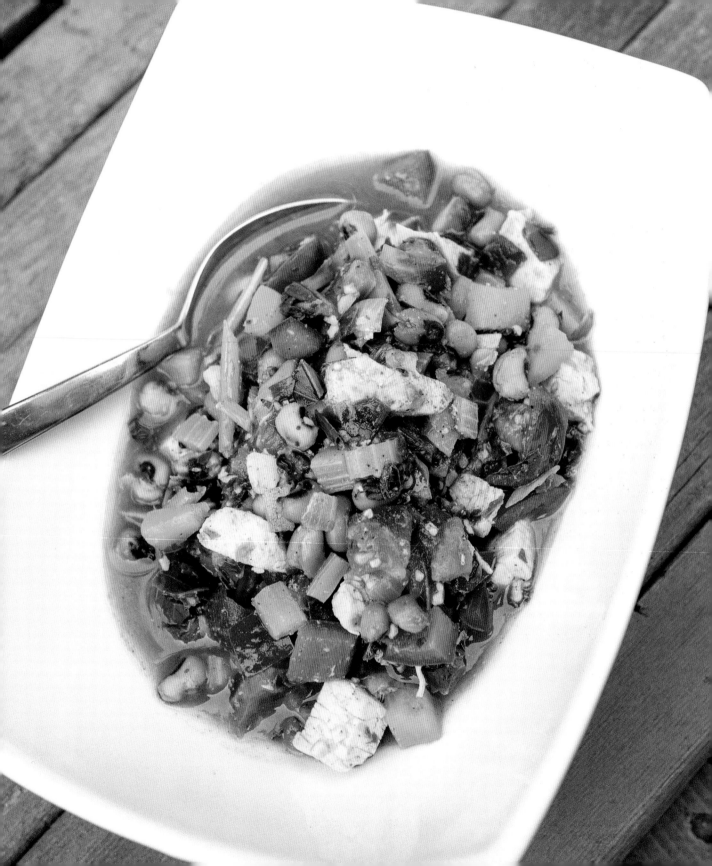

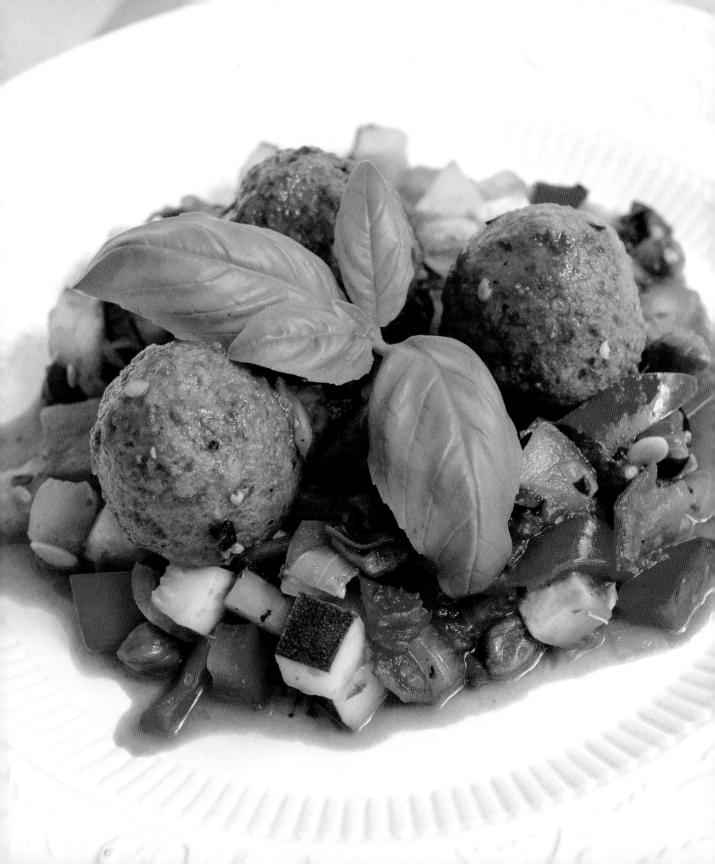

OVEN-ROASTED MEATBALLS WITH VEGETABLE CAPONATA

Oven-crisped meatballs find a juicy home in this hearty, chunky, Italian vegetable stew. Once baked and cooled, extra meatballs can be stored, tightly covered, in the freezer until needed.

YIELD: 6 CUPS (1.4 L) | SERVINGS: 4 | SERVING SIZE: 3 MEATBALLS + 1 ½ CUPS (350 ML) CAPONATA

MEATBALLS

1 lb (450 g) extra-lean ground beef

¼ cup (30 g) oat flour, whole grain

¼ cup (38 g) yellow onion, peeled, chopped small

1 tbsp (3 g) Italian flat-leaf parsley

1 tbsp (15 ml) fat-free milk

2 garlic cloves, peeled, minced

1 tsp ground black pepper

¼ tsp crushed red pepper flakes

2 large egg whites, lightly beaten with a fork

CAPONATA

2 tsp (10 ml) avocado oil

2 cups (300 g) yellow onion, chopped medium

4 garlic cloves, peeled, minced

1 tsp dried oregano leaves

½ tsp crushed red pepper flakes

¼ tsp sea salt (optional)

2 cups (164 g) eggplant, chopped medium

2 cups (220 g) zucchini, chopped medium

1 cup (175 g) red bell pepper, chopped medium

1 cup (140 g) yellow squash, chopped medium

1 cup (238 g) fat-free, low-sodium vegetable broth

2 cups (360 g) red ripe tomatoes, chopped

1 tbsp (11 g) kalamata olives, pitted, chopped

½ cup (20 g) Italian flat-leaf parsley, chopped

½ cup (12 g) fresh basil leaves

2 tsp (10 ml) extra virgin olive oil

½ tsp ground black pepper

1 tbsp (9 g) caper berries, drained

In a medium bowl, use your hands or a spoon to gently combine the meatball ingredients except for the egg whites. Be careful not to overwork the mixture, or it will become too dense and the meatballs will be too heavy. Gently work in the egg whites.

Shape into 12 individual ½-inch (1.3-cm) balls. Transfer to a sheet tray.

Preheat the oven broiler. Broil the meatballs about 4 inches (10 cm) from the heat for about 15 minutes or until tops are browned. Turn over and broil for another 15 minutes or until the meatballs are browned on the outside and no longer pink in the center. Place cooked meatballs onto paper towels to drain. Set aside until needed.

In a large heavy-bottomed pot, heat the oil over medium heat. Add the onions, garlic, oregano, pepper flakes and salt (optional). Cook, stirring occasionally for about 4 minutes. Add the eggplant and cook for about 4 minutes, stirring occasionally. Stir in the zucchini, bell pepper, squash and broth to combine.

Cover the pot and cook until the vegetables are tender, about 8 minutes, stirring half-way through.

Uncover the pot and stir in the tomatoes, olives, parsley, basil, olive oil, black pepper and capers. Stir the meatballs into the sauce to coat and cook another 2 minutes.

Place 3 meatballs on each plate and divide sauce evenly over the meatballs. If not eating immediately, cool completely before storing, tightly covered, in the refrigerator until ready to use.

NUTRITION (PER SERVING)
Calories 290, Total Fat 11 g, Saturated Fat 3 g, Trans Fat 0 g, Cholesterol 55 mg, Sodium 390 mg, Total Carbohydrate 24 g, Dietary Fiber 7 g, Sugars 11 g, Protein 26 g, Vitamin A 60%, Vitamin C 160%, Calcium 10%, Iron 25%

PAN-SEARED BEEF TENDERLOIN WITH SHIITAKES, LEMON AND PARSLEY

Shiitakes are the subtle star of this easy-to-execute dish. Lemon and parsley only enhance their umami flavor So delicious and elegant, you'll give your kitchen a five-star rating!

YIELD: 4 | SERVINGS: 4 | SERVING SIZE: 3 OUNCES (85 G) STEAK + ¾ CUP (44 G) MUSHROOMS

1 lb (450 g) beef tenderloin, trimmed of all visible fat, and cut into 4-oz (113-g) steaks

¼ tsp sea salt (optional)

½ tsp ground black pepper

2 tsp (10 ml) avocado oil, divided

3 cups (177 g) shiitake mushrooms, stems off, caps sliced

4 garlic cloves, peeled, minced

2 tbsp (20 g) shallot, peeled, minced

¼ cup (59 ml) dry white wine

¾ cup (178 ml) fat-free, low-sodium chicken stock

2 tbsp (30 ml) fresh lemon juice

2 tsp (10 ml) extra virgin olive oil

1 tbsp (3 g) Italian flat-leaf parsley leaves, chopped

Season both sides of the beef tenderloin steaks with sea salt (optional) and black pepper.

Heat 1 teaspoon avocado oil in a large heavy-bottomed skillet over medium-high heat. Add the beef tenderloin medallions, and cook approximately 5 minutes, turning halfway through or until desired doneness. Beef should be browned on both sides. Transfer the steaks to a plate and set aside until needed.

Still over medium-high heat, add the other 1 teaspoon of avocado oil and swirl to coat the pan. Add the shiitake mushrooms, garlic and shallots, and cook until the mushrooms are just tender, about 4 minutes, stirring frequently.

Add the white wine, chicken stock and lemon juice, and simmer until liquid is reduced by half, about 4 minutes.

Return the steaks to the pan, and allow them to cook for 1 minute, turning occasionally. Finish by adding the olive oil and parsley and stirring to combine.

Divide the medallions between 4 plates and top with the shiitake mixture. If not eating immediately, cool completely before storing, tightly covered, in the refrigerator.

NUTRITION (PER SERVING)

Calories 290, Total Fat 13 g, Saturated Fat 3.5 g, Trans Fat 0 g, Cholesterol 70 mg, Sodium 230 mg, Total Carbohydrate 13 g, Dietary Fiber 4 g, Sugars 4 g, Protein 29 g, Vitamin A 2%, Vitamin C 10%, Calcium 2%, Iron 15%

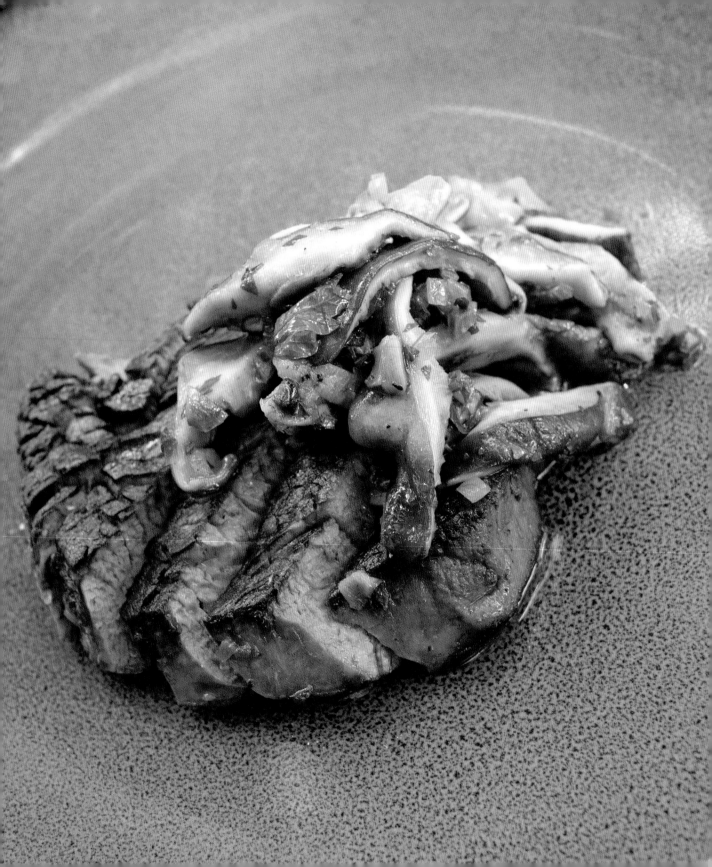

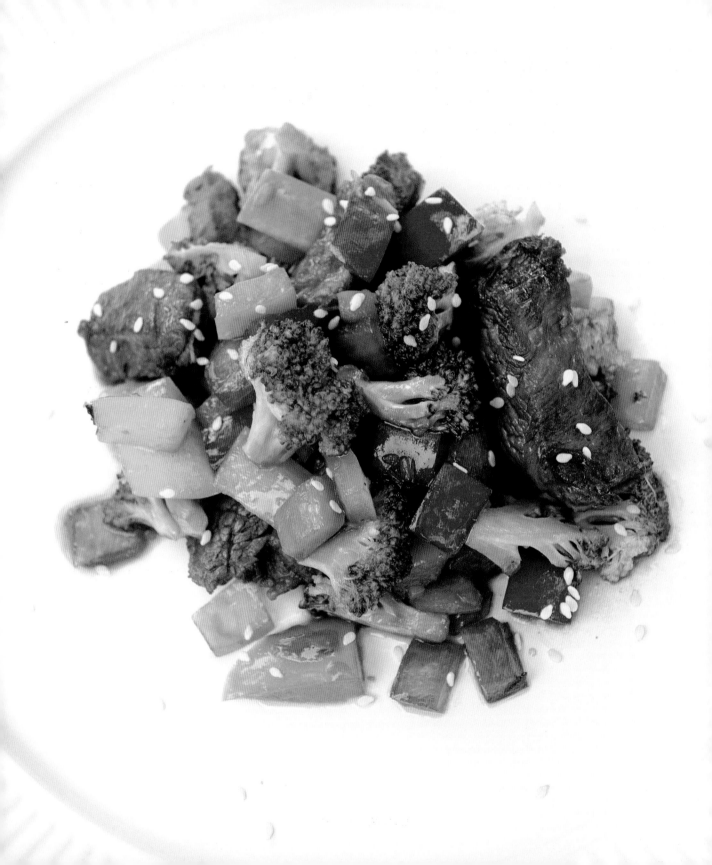

RAINBOW BEEF STIR-FRY

Stir-fry is a healthy cooking method that uses little added fat to get the job done. And with the rainbow of colorful vegetables, you may just find a pot of gold (or at least good health) at the bottom of your bowl.

YIELD: 4 | SERVINGS: 4 | SERVING SIZE: 1 ½ CUP (350 G)

2 tsp (5 g) fresh ginger root, minced

2 garlic cloves, peeled, minced

2 tbsp (12 g) scallion, white part only, thinly sliced

1 lb (450 g) boneless top sirloin steak, trimmed of all visible fat, cut into ¼-inch (6-mm) strips

1 cup (238 g) fat-free, low-sodium beef or chicken broth

2 tbsp (30 ml) low-sodium soy sauce

1 tsp toasted sesame oil

¼ tsp crushed red pepper flakes

1 tsp avocado oil

3 cups (213 g) broccoli florets, chopped medium

1 cup (175 g) red bell pepper, seeded, chopped medium

1 cup (175 g) yellow bell pepper, seeded, chopped medium

1 cup (175 g) orange bell pepper, seeded, chopped medium

1 cup (160 g) red onion, chopped medium

½ tsp ground black pepper

In a medium bowl, stir together the ginger root, garlic and scallions. Add the beef strips, turning to coat evenly. Cover and refrigerate for at least 30 minutes.

In a small bowl, whisk together the broth, soy sauce, sesame oil and red pepper flakes until combined. Set aside until needed.

In a large nonstick skillet or wok, heat the avocado oil over medium-high heat. Tip the skillet or wok to allow the oil to coat the bottom. Cook the beef for 5 minutes, stirring constantly. Transfer the beef to a side plate. The beef is only partially cooked at this point.

In the same skillet or wok, cook the broccoli, bell pepper and onions over medium-high heat for about 3 minutes or until just tender crisp.

Stir in the broth mixture. Bring to a simmer. Reduce the heat and simmer for 3 minutes or until reduced by half, stirring occasionally.

Stir in the beef and black pepper and cook for another 3 minutes or until the beef reaches desired doneness, stirring frequently.

NUTRITION (PER SERVING)
Calories 300, Total Fat 9 g, Saturated Fat 2.5 g, Trans Fat 0 g, Cholesterol 90 mg, Sodium 370 mg, Total Carbohydrate 18 g, Dietary Fiber 3 g, Sugars 5 g, Protein 40 g, Vitamin A 80%, Vitamin C 530%, Calcium 6%, Iron 25%

SANGRIA SALMON

Simple pan-seared salmon gets elevated by a complex, but not complicated, fresh citrus red wine sauce. Not a fan of salmon? Don't hesitate to use arctic char as a suitable alternative.

YIELD: 4 | SERVINGS: 4 | SERVING SIZE: 3 OUNCES SALMON (86 G) + ½ CUP SPINACH (15 G) + ½ CUP (119 ML) BROTH

- -

1 lb (454 g) wild salmon fillet, skin off, cut into 4-oz (113-g) medallions

1 tsp ground black pepper

4 tsp (20 ml) avocado oil, divided

2 garlic cloves, peeled, minced

¾ cup (120 g) red onion, peeled, sliced thin

1 ¼ cups (39 g) red ripe tomatoes, cut into wedges

½ cup (50 g) scallion, chopped

4 fresh orange segments

8 fresh lime segments

8 fresh lemon segments

4 fresh grapefruit segments

1 cup (237 ml) dry red wine (Cabernet)

1 tsp 100% pure honey

¼ tsp sea salt (optional)

2 tbsp (30 ml) balsamic vinegar

¼ cup (10 g) fresh basil leaves, chopped

6 cups (180 g) baby spinach

Dust the tops of the salmon fillets with the black pepper. Heat a large nonstick skillet over medium-high heat. Add the salmon fillets to the pan and cook for about 3 minutes on each side or until fully cooked throughout. Transfer the salmon to a plate until needed.

Still over medium-high heat, heat 2 teaspoons (10 ml) of oil. Add the garlic and onion, and cook, stirring occasionally for about 3 minutes until the onions are just starting to soften. Add the tomatoes, scallion and fruit segments, and stir to combine.

Add the red wine, honey, salt (optional) and balsamic vinegar, and cook until the liquid is reduced by half, about 4 minutes. Add the basil leaves, stirring to combine, and remove from the heat until needed.

In a separate large nonstick skillet, heat the remaining 2 teaspoons (10 ml) of oil over medium-high heat. Add the spinach, stirring constantly until it is wilted, about 2 minutes.

Divide the spinach among 4 shallow bowls. Top each with a salmon fillet. Divide the sangria reduction among the 4 bowls. If not eating immediately, cool thoroughly and store, tightly covered, in the refrigerator until ready to use.

- -

NUTRITION (PER SERVING)
Calories 320, Total Fat 12 g, Saturated Fat 1.5 g, Trans Fat 0 g, Cholesterol 60 mg, Sodium 240 mg, Total Carbohydrate 19 g, Dietary Fiber 4 g, Sugars 10 g, Protein 25 g, Vitamin A 100%, Vitamin C 100%, Calcium 10%, Iron 15%

- -

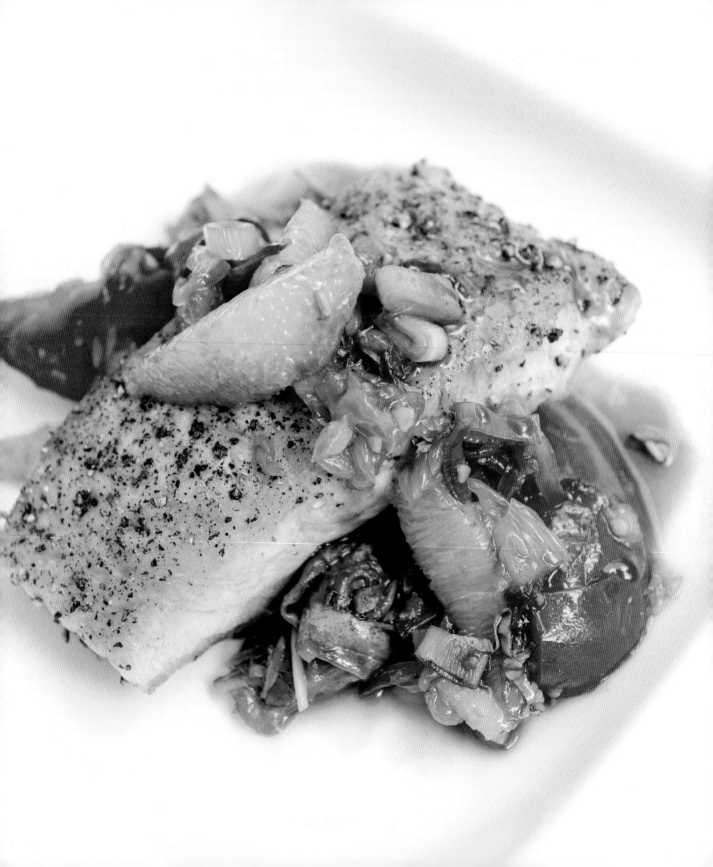

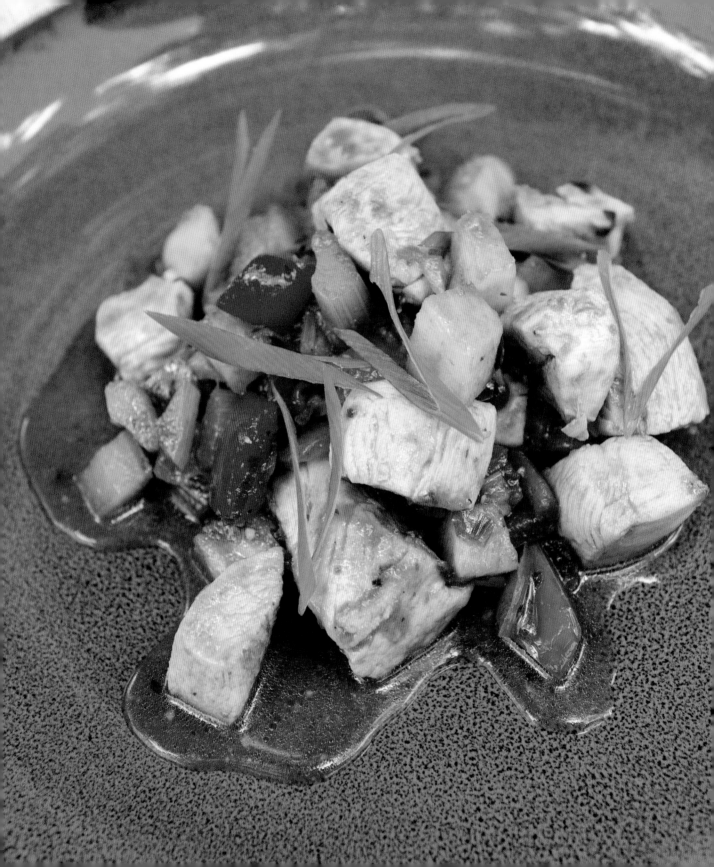

SEMISWEET & SOUR CHICKEN

Tender chunks of chicken, colorful Asian vegetables and a semi-sweet sauce make for an easy, less-sugary version of this take-out menu classic. Leftovers, if there are any, make for a great lunch the next day!

YIELD: 7 CUPS (1.5 L) | SERVINGS: 4 | SERVING SIZE: 1 ¾ CUPS (414 G)

1 tbsp (15 ml) avocado oil, divided

1 lb (454 g) chicken breast, boneless, skinless, trimmed of any visible fat, cut into 1-inch (2.5-cm) pieces

3 garlic clove

2 tsp (4 g) fresh ginger, minced

¼ tsp crushed red chili flakes

½ cup (50 g) scallion, white and green parts, chopped small

1 cup (150 g) onion, peeled, chopped medium

1 cup (101 g) celery, chopped medium

1 cup (128 g) carrot, peeled, chopped medium

1 cup (175 g) red bell pepper, seeded, chopped medium

1 cup (175 g) green bell pepper, seeded, chopped medium

½ cup (119 ml) dry white wine

2 tbsp (30 ml) plain rice vinegar

1 cup (238 ml) fat-free, low-sodium chicken stock

½ cup (113 ml) all-natural tomato sauce

2 tsp (10 ml) 100% pure honey

½ cup (83 g) fresh pineapple, peeled, chopped medium

1 tbsp (15 ml) fresh lime juice

2 tsp (10 ml) sesame oil

2 tbsp (6 g) fresh cilantro leaves, chopped

In a heavy-bottomed pot, heat 2 teaspoons (10 ml) oil over medium heat. Add the chicken and cook, stirring regularly, for 5 minutes. The chicken will not be done at this point. Transfer the chicken from the pot to a plate until needed. Drain the pot and discard any liquid from the chicken.

Return the pot to the stove, and still over medium heat, heat the remaining teaspoon of oil. Add the garlic, ginger, chili flakes and scallion, and cook, stirring occasionally, for 2 minutes.

Add the onion, celery, carrot, red bell pepper and green bell pepper, and cook for about 4 minutes, stirring occasionally or until the celery is tender crisp

Add the white wine, vinegar, chicken stock, tomato sauce, honey and pineapple, and stir to combine.

Return the chicken to the pot and cook covered over a simmer for about 15 minutes, until the chicken is fully cooked or reads an internal temperature of 165°F (74°C) with an instant-read thermometer.

Add the lime juice, sesame oil and cilantro leaves and stir to combine.

NUTRITION (PER SERVING)
Calories 300, Total Fat 10 g, Saturated Fat 1.5 g, Trans Fat 0 g, Cholesterol 90 mg, Sodium 140 mg, Total Carbohydrate 19 g, Dietary Fiber 3 g, Sugars 11 g, Protein 29 g, Vitamin A 140%, Vitamin C 130%, Calcium 6%, Iron 8%

SLOPPY (DOCTOR) JOES

A nod to the good Doctor with this still-sloppy yet healthy and sophisticated twist on the American classic. With a meaty portobella for the base, no bun needed or missed!

YIELD: 4 CUPS (1 L) | SERVINGS: 4 | SERVING SIZE: 1 CUP (237 ML) MIX + 1 MUSHROOM

- -

4 medium-sized portabella mushrooms, stems off

2 tbsp (30 ml) avocado oil, divided

1 lb (454 g) lean ground turkey

1 cup (150 g) onion, peeled, chopped small

2 garlic cloves, peeled, minced

1 cup (175 g) red bell pepper, seeded, chopped small

1 cup (110 g) carrots, peeled, grated

1 cup (110 g) zucchini, grated

½ cup (113 ml) all-natural tomato sauce

½ cup (119 ml) fat-free, low-sodium chicken stock

1 tbsp (15 ml) apple cider vinegar

2 tsp (2 g) chipotle in adobo

1 tsp low-sodium Worcestershire sauce

1 tsp ground black pepper

1 tbsp (3 g) fresh cilantro leaves, chopped

Preheat the oven to 375°F (190°C). Place the mushrooms, gill side up, on a baking sheet. Brush the tops evenly with 1 tablespoon (15 ml) of the avocado oil. Place in the oven on the middle rack and roast for approximately 30 minutes or until the mushrooms start to release their liquid and are tender soft. Remove from the oven, cover to keep warm, and set aside until needed.

In a large skillet heat the remaining 1 tablespoon (15 ml) of avocado oil over medium heat. Add the ground turkey, onion, garlic, red bell pepper and carrots, and sauté for about 8 to 10 minutes or until the turkey is cooked thoroughly and no pink is visible. Add the zucchini and stir to combine.

Add the tomato sauce, chicken stock, vinegar, chipotle, Worcestershire sauce and black pepper, and stir to combine. Place the portabellas, gill side up, upon the mix. Cook on a simmer, stirring occasionally until the liquid is reduced by at least half, and the mixture resembles a more tightly formed mix.

Add the cilantro and stir to combine.

Place one portabella on each of 4 plates. Divide the remaining Sloppy (Doctor) Joe mix evenly on top of the mushrooms. If not eating immediately, cool completely and store, tightly covered, in the refrigerator until ready to use.

- -

NUTRITION (PER SERVING)

Calories 320, Total Fat 18 g, Saturated Fat 3.5 g, Trans Fat 0 g, Cholesterol 90 mg, Sodium 190 mg, Total Carbohydrate 15 g, Dietary Fiber 4 g, Sugars 8 g, Protein 27 g, Vitamin A 140%, Vitamin C 100%, Calcium 6%, Iron 15%

- -

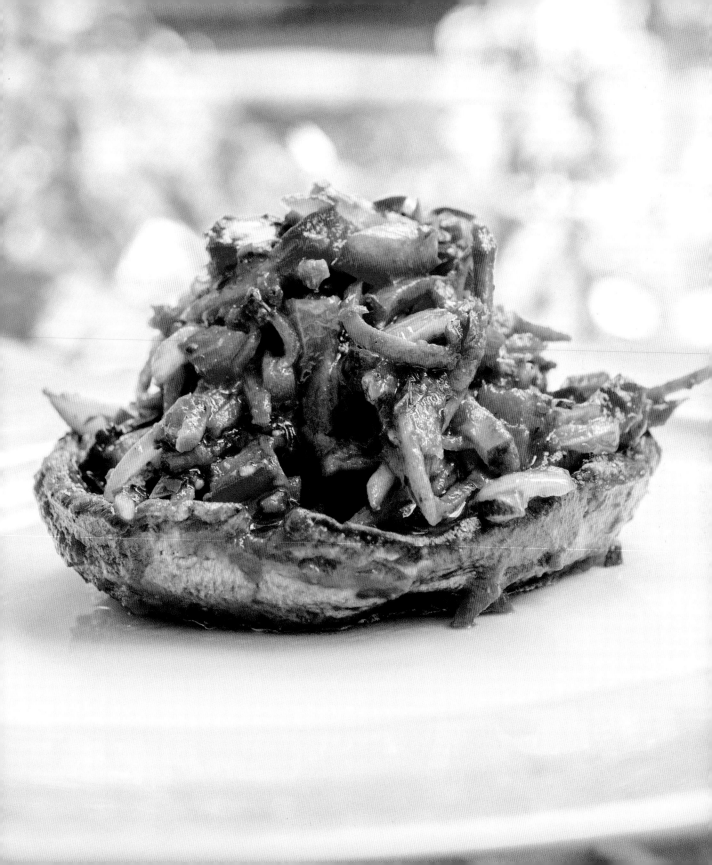

SMOKE-SIGNAL BUFFALO CHILI

Just as easy to make with lean ground beef or turkey, this warm chunky one-pot dish will have smoke coming out of your ears! To dial down the number of alarms, scale back on the chipotle, substitute smoked paprika and/or add extra yogurt to cool things off.

YIELD: 4 CUPS (1 L) | **SERVINGS: 4** | **SERVING SIZE: 1 CUP (113 G) + 1 TABLESPOON EACH CHEESE (8 G) AND YOGURT (15 G)**

2 tsp (10 ml) avocado oil, divided

1 lb (454 g) ground buffalo round

1 cup (150 g) yellow onion, chopped small

5 garlic cloves, minced

1 cup (100 g) scallion, white and green parts, chopped small

2 tbsp (15 g) chili powder

1 tbsp (16 g) ground cumin

1 ½ tsp (1 g) dried oregano

½ tsp ground black pepper

½ tsp sea salt (optional)

2 cups (476 ml) fat-free, low-sodium chicken broth

2 cups (360 g) red ripe tomatoes, chopped small

½ cup (65 g) roasted red pepper, chopped small

1 tbsp (15 ml) 100% pure honey

1 tbsp (16 g) tomato paste

1 tbsp (15 g) chipotle chillies in adobo, minced

2 tbsp (30 ml) fresh lime juice

¼ cup (13 g) fresh cilantro, chopped

¼ cup (61 g) plain fat-free Greek yogurt (optional)

¼ cup (28 g) reduced-fat shredded cheddar cheese (optional)

Heat 1 teaspoon of oil in a large heavy-bottomed soup pot on medium heat. Add the buffalo and sauté for about 5 minutes, breaking up the meat with a spoon, until cooked through. Transfer the meat with a slotted spoon to a separate plate. Set aside until needed.

Pour off and discard any liquid from the pot and add the other 1 teaspoon of oil. Add the onion and cook for about 1 minute until softened. Add the garlic and scallion and cook 1 minute more. Add the chili powder, cumin, oregano, black pepper and salt (optional), and stir to combine.

Add the chicken stock to the pot and simmer for about 5 minutes. Return the buffalo to the pot and add the tomatoes, roasted red pepper, honey, tomato paste and chipotle peppers. Bring to a boil, reduce the heat to a simmer and cook for about 30 minutes, stirring occasionally. Add water as needed if the chili begins to get too dry.

Stir in the lime juice and cilantro to combine.

Divide the chili into 4 bowls. Top each bowl with 1 tablespoon (15 g) of yogurt and cheddar cheese (8 g). If not using immediately, cool the chili completely before storing it tightly covered in the refrigerator.

NUTRITION (PER SERVING)

Calories 340, Total Fat 15 g, Saturated Fat 5 g, Trans Fat 0 g, Cholesterol 85 mg, Sodium 550 mg, Total Carbohydrate 19 g, Dietary Fiber 4 g, Sugars 11 g, Protein 36 g, Vitamin A 60%, Vitamin C 90%, Calcium 15%, Iron 15%

TURKEY JERKY KABOBS WITH CUCUMBER-DILL SAUCE

Island flavors spice up these balanced "meals on a stick" only to be cooled off by a sweet and tangy yogurt sauce. Leftover sauce? Pair with fresh cut vegetables for an easy refreshing snack.

YIELD: 8 KABOBS + 1 CUP (237 ML) SAUCE | SERVINGS: 4 | SERVING SIZE: 2 KABOBS + ¼ CUP (59 ML) SAUCE

1 tsp garlic powder

½ tsp cayenne pepper

1 tsp onion powder

½ tsp dried thyme leaves

¼ tsp sea salt (optional)

1 tsp ground black pepper, divided

¼ tsp ground nutmeg

¼ tsp ground cinnamon

1 cup (245 g) plain fat-free Greek yogurt

½ cup (75 g) cucumber, peel on, seeded, chopped small

1 tsp extra virgin olive oil

½ tsp red wine vinegar

1 tsp lemon juice

1 garlic clove, peeled, minced

2 tsp (2 g) fresh dill

1 lb (454 g) turkey tenderloin, trimmed of any visible fat, cut into 1 ½-inch (3.8-cm) cubes

1 tsp avocado oil

1 ½ cups (265 g) orange bell pepper, seeded, cut into 2-inch (5-cm) cubes

1 ½ cups (265 g) yellow pepper, seeded, cut into 2-inch (5-cm) cubes

2 cups (298 g) cherry tomatoes, whole

2 cups (320 g) red onion, peeled, cut into 2-inch (5-cm) cubes

In a medium bowl, mix together the garlic powder, cayenne, onion powder, thyme leaves, salt (optional), ½ teaspoon black pepper, nutmeg and cinnamon. Set aside until needed.

In a medium bowl, combine the yogurt, cucumber, ½ teaspoon black pepper, olive oil, red wine vinegar, lemon juice, fresh garlic and dill. Stir to combine. Store the sauce in the refrigerator until needed.

On 8-inch (20-cm) metal or water-soaked bamboo skewers, alternately skewer a piece of turkey, pepper, cherry tomato, piece of turkey, onion, pepper and turkey until all the turkey and vegetables are skewered. Place the kabobs on a baking sheet.

Brush the kabobs on all sides with the avocado oil. Sprinkle kabobs on all sides with the jerk seasoning mix to generously coat them.

Preheat the grill to medium. Place the kabobs on the grill grate on an angle. Cook for approximately 20 minutes or until there is no longer pink inside the turkey and the internal temperature registers 165°F (74°C) on an instant–read thermometer.

Remove the kabobs from the grill and place on each of 4 plates. Top with ¼ cup (59 ml) sauce. If not using immediately, cool completely and store tightly covered in the refrigerator until ready to use.

NUTRITION (PER SERVING)

Calories 310, Total Fat 11 g, Saturated Fat 2.5 g, Trans Fat 0 g, Cholesterol 75 mg, Sodium 240 mg, Total Carbohydrate 19 g, Dietary Fiber 5 g, Sugars 11 g, Protein 32 g, Vitamin A 80%, Vitamin C 260%, Calcium 10%, Iron 15%

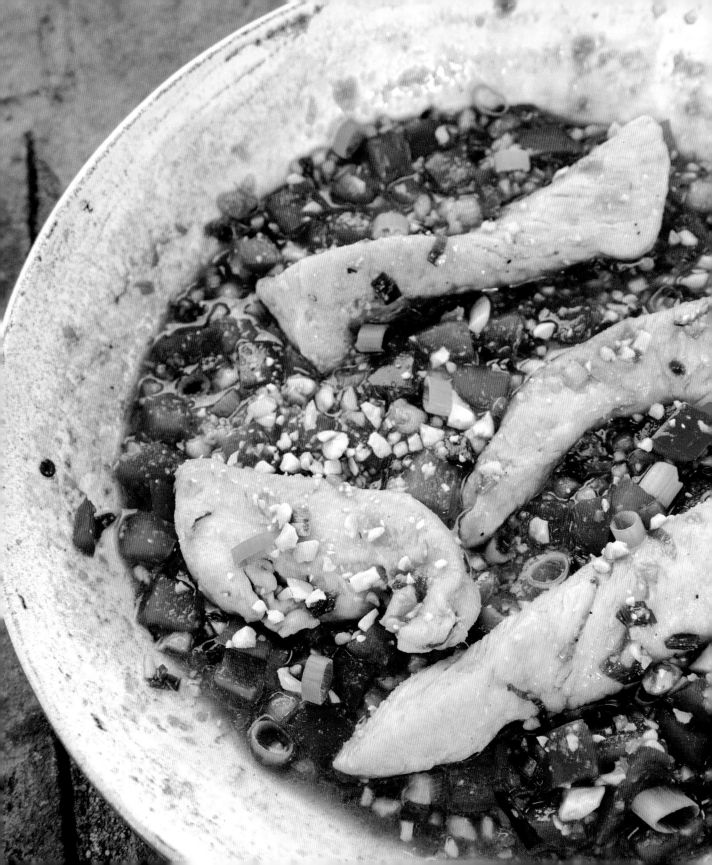

SUPERFAST CHICKEN & CASHEWS

For those who never have enough time for a healthy supper, this is the high-speed go-to you've been searching for. Superfast can still be super healthy!

YIELD: 6 CUPS (1.5 L) | SERVINGS: 4 | SERVING SIZE: 1 ½ CUPS (355 G)

1 tbsp (15 ml) avocado oil

1 lb (454 g) chicken breast tenderloins, boneless, skinless, trimmed of all visible fat, cut in half

2 cups (350 g) red bell pepper, seeded, chopped medium

½ cup (50 g) scallion, green and white parts, chopped medium

2 tsp (6 g) garlic powder

½ tsp ground ginger

½ tsp red hot sauce

1 tsp plain rice vinegar

2 tbsp (30 ml) low-sodium soy sauce

2 tbsp (30 ml) dry white wine

¼ cup (59 ml) fat-free, low-sodium chicken stock

½ cup (65 g) cashews, dry roasted, unsalted, chopped

Heat the oil in a large skillet or wok over medium-high heat. Add the chicken breast and cook for about 3 minutes until lightly browned.

Add the bell pepper, scallion, garlic powder and ground ginger. Stir to coat, and cook another 2 minutes until the peppers are just tender crisp.

Add the red hot sauce, rice vinegar, soy sauce, white wine and chicken stock, and cook until the liquid is reduced by half, about 4 minutes.

Fold in the cashews and stir to coat.

Divide evenly among 4 plates. If not eating immediately, cool completely and store, tightly covered, in the refrigerator until use.

NUTRITION (PER SERVING)

Calories 310, Total Fat 14 g, Saturated Fat 3 g, Trans Fat 0 g, Cholesterol 90 mg, Sodium 160 mg, Total Carbohydrate 13 g, Dietary Fiber 3 g, Sugars 5 g, Protein 30 g, Vitamin A 50%, Vitamin C 190%, Calcium 4%, Iron 15%

WALNUT-SAGE CRUSTED TROUT WITH GREEN BEANS

High in omega 3 fats, trout makes a great substitute if you find salmon's flavor a bit too strong. Walnuts and sage make for a crispy crust that balances out tender green beans.

YIELD: 4 | SERVINGS: 4 | SERVING SIZE: 2 FILLETS + 1 CUP (110 G) GREEN BEANS

½ cup (58 g) walnuts

1 tbsp (2 g) fresh sage

¼ tsp sea salt (optional)

¼ tsp ground black pepper

8 rainbow trout fillets, approximately 1 ¼ lbs (567 g)

1 tbsp (15 ml) Dijon mustard

4 cups (440 g) thin green beans

1 tsp avocado oil

2 garlic cloves, peeled, minced

1 tbsp (15 ml) fresh lemon juice

Preheat the oven to 350°F (180°C). In a food processor or blender, pulse the walnuts, sage, salt (optional) and black pepper until the sage is chopped and the walnuts reach a fine meal consistency. Set aside until needed.

Place the trout fillets flesh side up on a baking sheet. Brush the Dijon mustard over the trout fillets to coat.

Sprinkle the walnut-sage mix evenly over the top of the fillets.

In a separate medium bowl, toss the green beans with the oil and garlic. Place the green beans on another baking sheet or on the same sheet with the trout, if room is available.

Roast in the oven for approximately 15 minutes or until the trout is cooked fully and the green beans are just fork tender.

Remove the baking sheet from the oven and sprinkle the lemon juice over the green beans.

Divide the green beans evenly among 4 plates. Place 2 trout fillets on top of the green beans on each plate.

If not eating immediately, allow it to cool completely and store, tightly covered, in the refrigerator until ready to use.

NUTRITION (PER SERVING)
Calories 290, Total Fat 18 g, Saturated Fat 2.5 g, Trans Fat 0 g, Cholesterol 60 mg, Sodium 140 mg, Total Carbohydrate 11 g, Dietary Fiber 4 g, Sugars 4 g, Protein 24 g, Vitamin A 15%, Vitamin C 30%, Calcium 15%, Iron 10%

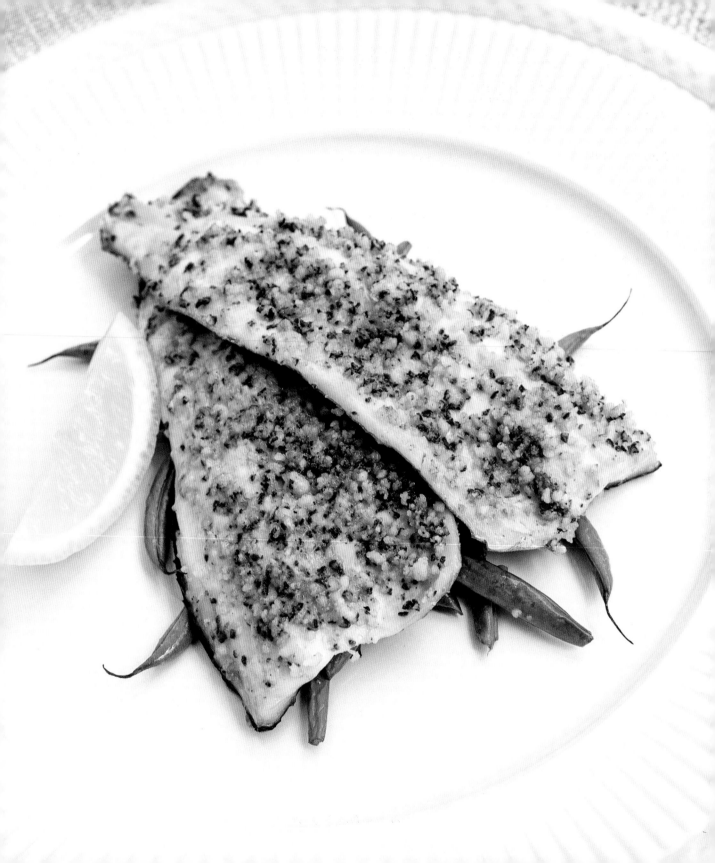

SALADS & SOUPS

Think lean and green isn't your thing? Think again! Wait until you taste these fast and fresh recipes, and see the results served with them! You'll be a believer in no time!

BAJA COBB SALAD
WITH AVOCADO-WASABI DRESSING

The classic Cobb with a fun California twist. Surf's up when this salad's served!

**YIELD: 2 SALADS | SERVINGS: 2 | SERVING SIZE: 1 SALAD + ¼ CUP (59 ML) DRESSING
DRESSING | YIELD: 2 CUPS (473 ML)**

- -

DRESSING

½ avocado, peeled, seeded

3 tsp (16 g) wasabi paste

¼ cup (59 ml) unseasoned rice vinegar

¼ cup (59 ml) cold water

¼ cup (59 ml) lemon juice

2 tsp (10 ml) 100% pure honey

¼ cup (59 ml) avocado oil

1 garlic clove, peeled

1 tbsp (3 g) fresh basil

1 tbsp (3 g) fresh cilantro

½ tsp ground black pepper

¼ tsp sea salt (optional)

SALAD

4 cups (188 g) romaine lettuce, chopped

3 oz (85 g) grilled chicken, chopped

2 hard-boiled eggs, quartered

1 tbsp (7 g) reduced-fat shredded Monterey Jack cheese

1 tbsp (7 g) reduced-fat shredded sharp cheddar cheese

½ cup (75 g) cherry tomatoes, halved

2 slices red onion, peeled

½ cup (55 g) shredded carrots, peeled

½ cup (50 g) red radish, trimmed, sliced thin

2 tsp (6 g) dry-roasted sunflower seeds

½ cup (115 g) fresh orange segments

Place all the dressing ingredients in a blender and blend until combined. Store covered in the refrigerator until ready to use.

In a large bowl, combine all the salad ingredients. If using both servings immediately, add ½ cup (118 ml) dressing and toss to coat. If using only one serving, add ¼ cup (59 ml) dressing and toss to coat. Store the remainder of the salad mix and dressing separately, tightly covered, in the refrigerator until ready to use.

- -

NUTRITION (PER SERVING)
Calories 200, Total Fat 14 g, Saturated Fat 2.5 g, Trans Fat 0 g, Cholesterol 50 mg, Sodium 290 mg, Total Carbohydrate 21 g, Dietary Fiber 6 g, Sugars 11 g, Protein 25 g, Vitamin A 270%, Vitamin C 80%, Calcium 15%, Iron 10%

- -

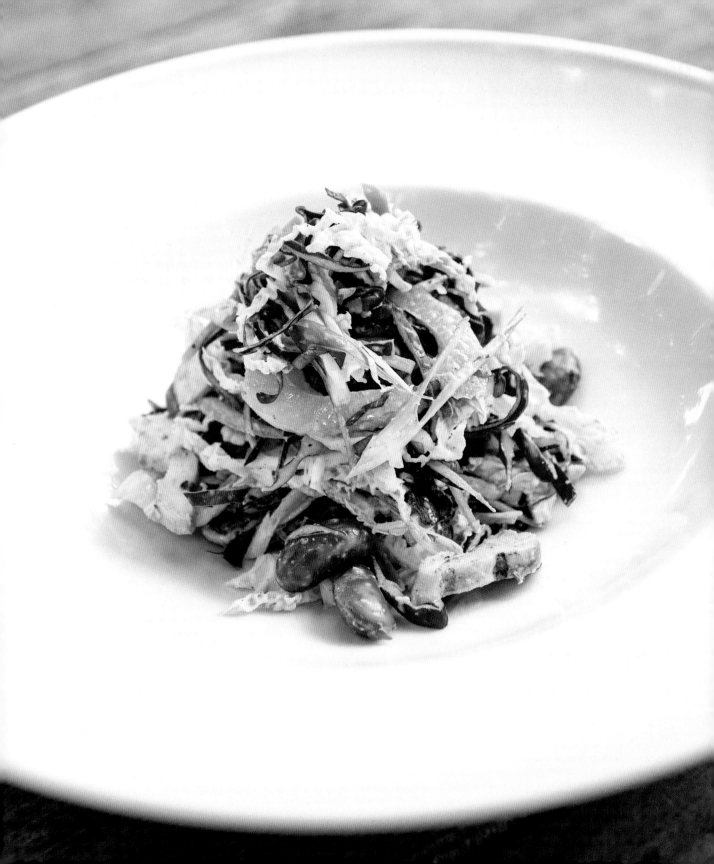

BBQ CHICKEN COLESLAW

Need something healthy but great-tasting to bring to a summer BBQ or get-together? This is the dish! Sure to be a creamy, crunchy and smoky hit.

YIELD: 2 SALADS | SERVINGS: 2 | SERVING SIZE: 1 SALAD + ¼ CUP (59 ML) DRESSING
DRESSING | YIELD: ABOUT 2 CUPS (473 ML)

DRESSING

¾ cup (184 g) plain fat-free Greek yogurt

¾ cup (177 ml) low-fat buttermilk

¼ cup (59 ml) apple cider vinegar

1 tbsp (15 ml) Dijon mustard

2 tsp (5 g) chili powder

2 tsp (6 g) garlic powder

2 tsp (5 g) onion powder

2 tsp (5 g) smoked paprika

1 tsp cumin

1 tsp black pepper

½ tsp cayenne pepper

½ tsp sea salt (optional)

SALAD

6-oz (170-g) grilled chicken, chopped

2 cups (140 g) green cabbage, shredded

1 cup (140 g) red cabbage, shredded

½ cup (55 g) carrots, peeled, shredded

½ cup (51 g) celery, sliced thin on the bias

½ cup (25 g) scallion, green part only, sliced thin on the bias

1 tbsp (7 g) pecans, dry-roasted, chopped

½ cup (92 g) red kidney beans, drained, rinsed

¼ cup (13 g) fresh cilantro leaves, chopped

Place all the dressing ingredients in the blender and blend to combine.

In a large bowl, combine all the salad ingredients. If using both servings immediately, add ½ cup (118 ml) dressing and toss to coat. If using only one serving, add ¼ cup (59 ml) dressing to serving and toss to coat. Store the remainder of the salad mix and dressing separately, tightly covered, in the refrigerator until ready to use.

NUTRITION (PER SERVING)

Calories 300, Total Fat 6 g, Saturated Fat 1.5 g, Trans Fat 0 g, Cholesterol 90 mg, Sodium 290 mg, Total Carbohydrate 27 g, Dietary Fiber 10 g, Sugars 9 g, Protein 36 g, Vitamin A 200%, Vitamin C 90%, Calcium 15%, Iron 15%

BUFFALO CHICKEN WEDGE WITH BUFFALO RANCH DRESSING

A mound of colorful, crisp vegetables, a tangy buffalo ranch dressing and easy, shredded rotisserie chicken will keep you from getting nutritionally "wedged" between a rock and a hard place.

YIELD: 2 SALADS | SERVINGS: 2 | SERVING SIZE: 1 SALAD + ¼ CUP (59 ML) DRESSING
DRESSING | YIELD 2 CUPS (473 ML)

- -

DRESSING

¾ cup (177 ml) low-fat buttermilk

1 cup (245 g) plain fat-free Greek yogurt

¼ cup (59 ml) hot sauce (I prefer Frank's RedHot Sauce)

4 tbsp (61 ml) avocado oil

1 tsp garlic powder

½ tsp black pepper

SALAD

½ head iceberg lettuce, cut in half lengthwise

6 oz (170 g) roasted chicken, shredded

1 cup (31 g) pear tomatoes, halved

½ cup (51 g) celery, sliced thin on the bias

½ cup (55 g) carrot, peeled, shredded

½ cup (25 g) scallion, green part only, sliced thin on the bias

2 slices red onion, peeled

¼ cup (28 g) reduced-fat shredded sharp cheddar cheese

½ avocado, sliced

Place all the dressing ingredients in a blender and blend until combined. Store covered in the refrigerator until ready to use.

In a large bowl, combine all the salad ingredients. If using both servings immediately, add ½ cup (118 ml) dressing and toss to coat. If using only one serving, add ¼ cup (59 ml) dressing to the serving and toss to coat. Store the remainder of the salad mix and dressing separately, tightly covered, in the refrigerator until ready to use.

- -

NUTRITION (PER SERVING)
Calories 340, Total Fat 4.5 g, Saturated Fat 2 g, Trans Fat 0 g, Cholesterol 95 mg, Sodium 470 mg, Total Carbohydrate 16 g, Dietary Fiber 4 g, Sugars 10 g, Protein 34 g, Vitamin A 130%, Vitamin C 35%, Calcium 20%, Iron 8%

- -

CURRIED CAULIFLOWER SOUP

Not all white foods are bad for us! Creamy cauliflower teams up with anti-inflammatory spices, lemon juice and fresh cilantro in this smooth puree. The sunny color and warm texture makes it a perfect choice for a rainy, cool day.

YIELD: 8 CUPS (2 L) | SERVINGS: 4 | SERVING SIZE: 2 CUPS (490 G) + 1 TABLESPOON (15 G) YOGURT

4 cups (400 g) cauliflower florets, chopped medium

1 cup (150 g) yellow onion, peeled, chopped medium

1 cup (128 g) carrot, peeled, chopped medium

½ cup (51 g) celery, chopped medium

1 fresh garlic clove, peeled, minced

1 tbsp (15 ml) avocado oil

1 ½ tbsp (9 g) curry powder

¼ tsp ground toasted coriander

½ tsp ground cumin

¼ tsp ground cinnamon

6 cups (1.5 L) fat-free, low-sodium chicken stock

2 tsp (10 ml) fresh lemon juice

1 tbsp (3 g) fresh cilantro

¼ tsp sea salt (optional)

¼ cup (61 g) plain fat-free Greek yogurt

Preheat the oven to 375°F (190°C). In a large bowl, mix the cauliflower florets, onion, carrot, celery and garlic with the avocado oil to coat. Spread evenly on a large baking sheet. Roast in the oven for about 25 minutes or until the vegetables are browned and just tender. Remove from the oven.

In a medium pot, heat the remainder of the oil over medium heat. Add the spices and cook, stirring often, for about 1 minute.

Carefully add the vegetables, chicken stock and lemon juice. Cook until the liquid is reduced by half, about 4 minutes.

Add the cilantro and salt (optional) and stir to combine. In small batches, transfer the soup to a blender and carefully blend until smooth. Continue until all the soup is puréed.

Serve the soup in bowls garnished with 1 tablespoon (15 g) of yogurt.

NUTRITION (PER SERVING)

Calories 130, Total Fat 4.5 g, Saturated Fat 0.5 g, Trans Fat 0 g, Cholesterol less than 5 mg, Sodium 340 mg, Total Carbohydrate 14 g, Dietary Fiber 5 g, Sugars 6 g, Protein 10 g, Vitamin A 110%, Vitamin C 90%, Calcium 10%, Iron 8%

GREEK GOD SALAD
WITH RED WINE VINAIGRETTE

We can't swear that Hercules himself dined on this salad, but it's sure to give any mere mortal the nutritional goods to be godly (healthy, that is)!

YIELD: 2 SALADS | SERVINGS: 2 | SERVING SIZE: 1 SALAD + ¼ CUP (59 ML) DRESSING
DRESSING | YIELD: ABOUT 2 CUPS (473 ML)

DRESSING

¼ cup (25 g) scallion, white part, minced

1 tbsp (2 g) dried oregano

2 garlic cloves, peeled, minced

½ tsp black pepper

1 tsp Dijon mustard

1 ¼ cups (296 ml) red wine vinegar

½ cup (120 ml) extra virgin olive oil

SALAD

4 cups (188 g) romaine lettuce, rough chopped

6 oz (170 g) grilled chicken, chopped

½ cup (52 g) English cucumber, peel on, sliced thin

½ cup (90 g) red ripe tomatoes, chopped

½ cup (84 g) canned artichokes, drained, pressed

½ cup (65 g) roasted red peppers, drained, rinsed

6 pitted kalamata olives, chopped

2 slices red onion, peeled

1 scallion, green part, sliced thin on the bias

2 tbsp (19 g) reduced-fat feta cheese

Place all the dressing ingredients except the extra virgin olive oil in a small bowl. Gradually whisk in the olive oil until emulsified. Keep the unused dressing covered tightly in the refrigerator. Shake well before using.

In a large bowl, combine all the salad ingredients. If using both servings immediately, add ½ cup (118 ml) dressing and toss to coat. If using only one serving, add ¼ cup (59 ml) dressing and toss to coat. Store the remainder of the salad mix and dressing separately, tightly covered, in the refrigerator until ready to use.

NUTRITION (PER SERVING)

Calories 380, Total Fat 21 g, Saturated Fat 4 g, Trans Fat 0 g, Cholesterol 90 mg, Sodium 490 mg, Total Carbohydrate 18 g, Dietary Fiber 8 g, Sugars 6 g, Protein 32 g, Vitamin A 200%, Vitamin C 110%, Calcium 8%, Iron 15%

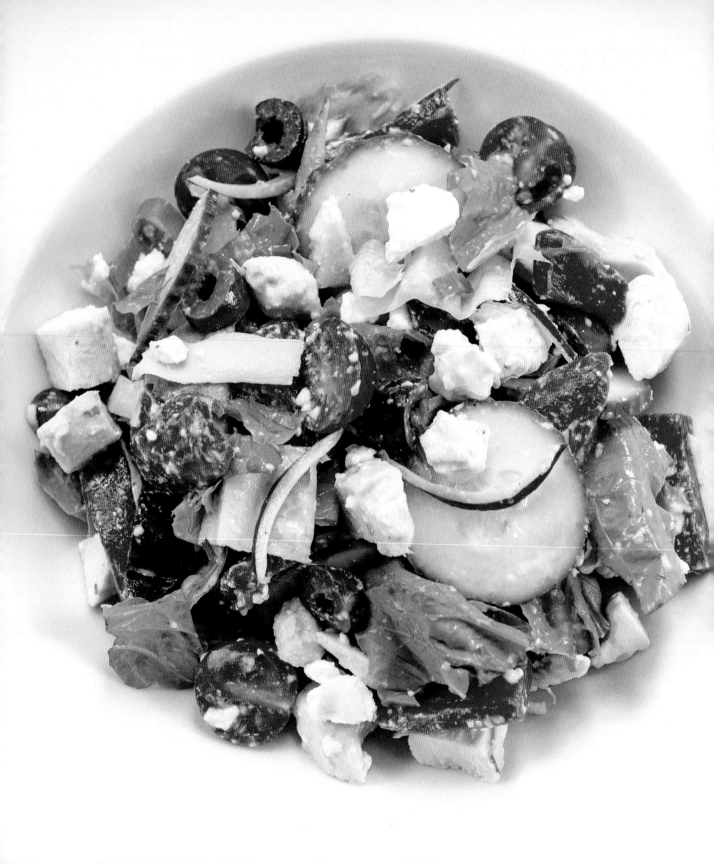

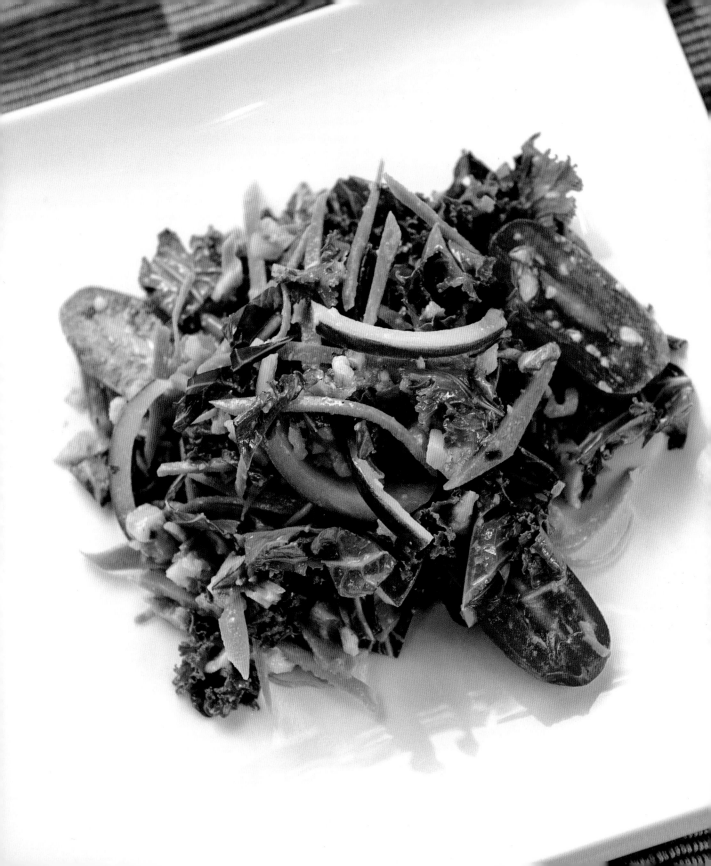

KILLER KALE SALAD
WITH ROASTED GARLIC VINAIGRETTE

Smoky grilled chicken, nutty walnuts and a garlicky lemon dressing stand up nicely to hearty kale. After the first bite you'll be "dying" for more!

YIELD: 2 SALADS | SERVINGS: 2 | SERVING SIZE: 1 SALAD + ¼ CUP (59 ML) DRESSING
DRESSING | YIELD: ABOUT 2 CUPS (473 ML)

DRESSING

1 head garlic, separated into cloves, peeled

1 tsp avocado oil

1 ¼ cups (296 ml) lemon juice

¼ tsp salt

¼ tsp black pepper

¼ tsp crushed red chili flakes

⅓ cup (78 ml) extra virgin olive oil

SALAD

2 cups (134 g) Italian kale, large tough stems discarded, chopped

2 cups (60 g) baby spinach

6 oz (170 g) grilled chicken, chopped

½ cup (55 g) shredded carrots

2 tbsp (14 g) walnuts, chopped

½ cup (25 g) scallions, green part only, slice thin on the bias

½ cup (75 g) pear tomatoes, halved

2 slices red onion, peeled

Preheat the oven to 400°F (204°C). Place the garlic cloves on a piece of tinfoil large enough to fold over. Drizzle with the avocado oil and toss to coat. Fold the tinfoil so edges are crimped closed.

Roast the garlic on the middle oven rack for about 35 minutes or until the cloves are softened and tender. Remove from the oven, open tinfoil carefully and allow it to cool completely.

In a small bowl, whisk together the cooled roasted garlic, lemon juice, salt, black pepper and red chili flakes until combined. Gradually whisk in the olive oil until combined. Keep the unused dressing covered tightly in the refrigerator. Shake well as needed before using.

In a large bowl, combine all the salad ingredients. If using both servings immediately, add ½ cup (118 ml) dressing and toss to coat. If using only one serving, add ¼ cup (59 ml) dressing to the serving and toss to coat. Store the remainder of the salad mix and dressing separately, tightly covered, in the refrigerator until ready to use.

NUTRITION (PER SERVING)
Calories 350, Total Fat 18 g, Saturated Fat 2.5 g, Trans Fat 0 g, Cholesterol 90 mg, Sodium 180 mg, Total Carbohydrate 19 g, Dietary Fiber 4 g, Sugars 5 g, Protein 32 g, Vitamin A 260%, Vitamin C 190%, Calcium 15%, Iron 15%

PASTALESS GRILLED-VEGETABLE PRIMAVERA SALAD WITH CREAMY ITALIAN DRESSING

With the smoky deep flavor of grilled chicken and seasonal vegetables, and a tangy, creamy vinaigrette to tie it all together, you won't even miss that other ingredient. What was it again? Exactly!

YIELD: 2 SALADS | SERVINGS: 2 | SERVING SIZE: 1 SALAD + ¼ CUP (59 ML) DRESSING
DRESSING | YIELD: ABOUT 2 CUPS (473 ML)

- -

DRESSING

1 cup (237 ml) red wine vinegar

1 cup (245 g) plain fat-free Greek yogurt

2 garlic cloves, peeled, minced

½ cup (50 g) scallion, all parts, chopped small

1 tbsp (3 g) fresh basil leaves

1 tbsp (3 g) fresh Italian parsley leaves

½ tsp ground black pepper

Dash sea salt (optional)

⅓ cup (78 ml) extra virgin olive oil

SALAD

2 medium portabella mushroom caps, whole

2 quarters red bell pepper, seeded, quartered

1 small zucchini, halved lengthwise

1 small yellow squash, halved lengthwise

1 small fennel bulb, quartered

1 tsp avocado oil

4 cups (400 g) seasonal mixed greens (mesclun mix)

3 oz (85 g) grilled chicken

½ cup (120 g) canned no-salt added chickpeas, drained, rinsed

10 green beans, whole

½ cup (90 g) red ripe tomatoes, chopped

½ cup (84 g) quartered artichoke hearts, drained

Place all the dressing ingredients except the olive oil in a small bowl. Gradually whisk in the olive oil until emulsified. Keep the unused dressing covered tightly in the refrigerator. Shake well as needed before using.

Preheat the grill to medium. In a large bowl, toss the mushrooms, bell pepper, zucchini, yellow squash and fennel bulb with the avocado oil. Grill each vegetable about 2–3 minutes on each side, or until just tender crisp. Remove from the grill and allow to cool before adding to salad.

In a large bowl, combine all the salad ingredients. If using both servings immediately, add ½ cup (118 ml) dressing and toss to coat. If using only one serving, add ¼ cup (59 ml) dressing to the serving and toss to coat. Store the remainder of the salad mix and dressing separately, tightly covered, in the refrigerator until ready to use.

- -

NUTRITION (PER SERVING)

Calories 360, Total Fat 15 g, Saturated Fat 2.5 g, Trans Fat 0 g, Cholesterol 90 mg, Sodium 220 mg, Total Carbohydrate 24 g, Dietary Fiber 10 g, Sugars 9 g, Protein 35 g, Vitamin A 140%, Vitamin C 160%, Calcium 10%, Iron 15%

- -

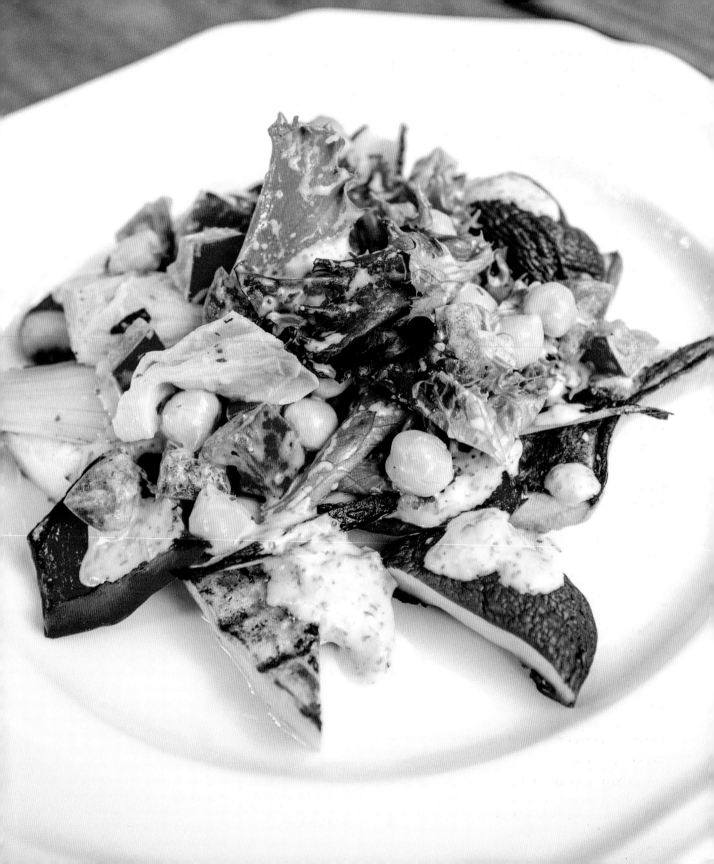

GAV-SPACHO

With a nod to Chef "Gav's" favorite home version, nothing beats these refreshing, seasonal and cool flavors on a hot summer day. Need a sauce for grilled chicken and fish, or a salsa dipper for garden fresh pepper strips? No problem. Gav-spacho to the rescue!

YIELD: 8 CUPS (2 L) | SERVINGS: 4 | SERVING SIZE: 2 CUPS (473 ML)

---

6 red ripe tomatoes, chopped medium

1 cucumber, peeled, seeded, chopped medium

1 red bell pepper, seeded,

3 garlic cloves, peeled, minced

3 cups (708 ml) low-sodium tomato juice

¼ cup (60 ml) extra virgin olive oil

3 tbsp (45 ml) apple cider vinegar

¼ cup (13 g) fresh cilantro leaves, chopped

1 lime, juiced

½ tsp ground cumin

¼ tsp sea salt (optional)

In a blender or food processor, combine all the ingredients until coarsely puréed.

Refrigerate, tightly covered, until chilled.

NUTRITION (PER SERVING)
Calories 230, Total Fat 14 g, Saturated Fat 2 g, Trans Fat 0 g, Cholesterol 0 mg, Sodium 290 mg, Total Carbohydrate 24 g, Dietary Fiber 6 g, Sugars 17 g, Protein 4 g, Vitamin A 130%, Vitamin C 230%, Calcium 6%, Iron 10%

PHILLY CHEESESTEAK SALAD WITH HORSEY SAUCE

Inspired by the City of Brotherly Love classic, there's no doubt the spicy horseradish dressing, shaved lean beef, rich cheeses and hearty vegetables will make this your new game-day favorite!

YIELD: 2 SALADS | SERVINGS: 2 | SERVING SIZE: 1 SALAD + ¼ CUP (59 ML) DRESSING
DRESSING | YIELD: ABOUT 2 CUPS (473 ML)

DRESSING

1 cup (121 g) fat-free sour cream

1 cup (245 g) plain fat-free Greek yogurt

4 tbsp (60 g) prepared horseradish

1 tsp lemon juice

1 tbsp (6 g) scallion, green part only, chopped small

½ tsp ground black pepper

Dash salt (optional)

SALAD

4 cups (188 g) romaine lettuce, chopped

6 oz (170 g) lean, shaved roast beef

½ cup (90 g) green bell pepper, sliced

½ cup (65 g) yellow onion, peeled, sliced

1 cup (59 g) cremini or brown button mushrooms, sliced

2 garlic cloves, peeled, minced

2 tsp (1 g) fresh rosemary, minced

1 tsp avocado oil

¼ cup (28 g) reduced-fat 4-cheese Italian blend shredded cheese

4 slices red ripe tomato

Place the dressing ingredients in a small bowl. Whisk together until combined. Keep the unused dressing covered tightly in the refrigerator. Shake well as needed before using.

In a large bowl, combine all the salad ingredients. If using both servings immediately, add ½ cup (118 ml) dressing and toss to coat. If using only one serving, add ¼ cup (59 ml) dressing and toss to coat. Store the remainder of the salad mix and dressing separately, tightly covered, in the refrigerator until ready to use.

NUTRITION (PER SERVING)
Calories 300, Total Fat 13 g, Saturated Fat 5 g, Trans Fat 0 g, Cholesterol 80 mg, Sodium 290 mg, Total Carbohydrate 16 g, Dietary Fiber 4 g, Sugars 8 g, Protein 30 g, Vitamin A 180%, Vitamin C 70%, Calcium 25%, Iron 20%

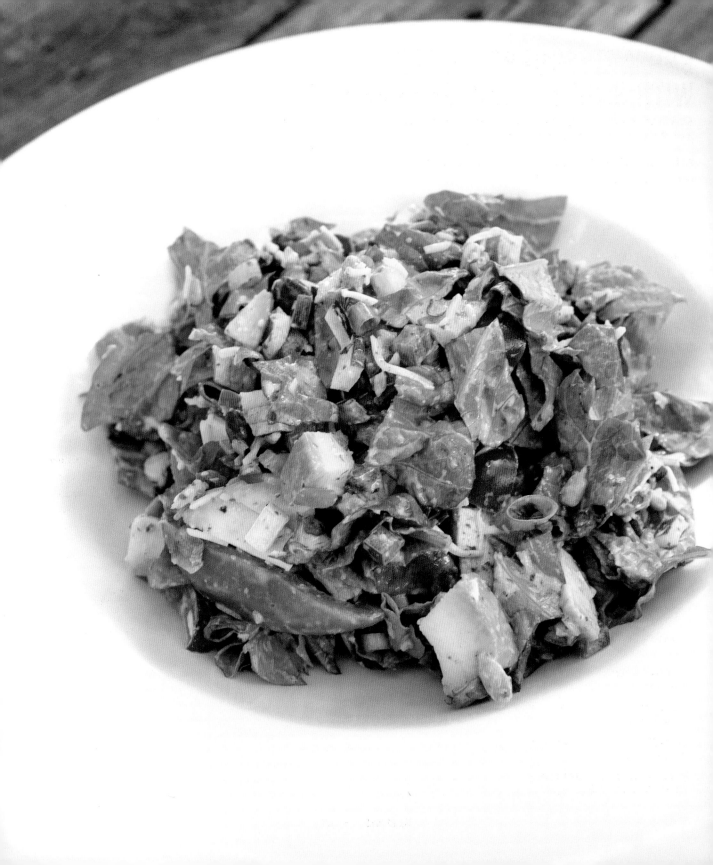

SANTA FE CHOPPED SALAD WITH SMOKY RANCH DRESSING

Small veggies means big flavor! There's something about chopping the veggies this size that makes them incredibly delicious. More veggies matters!

YIELD: 2 SALADS | SERVINGS: 2 | SERVING SIZE: 1 SALAD + ¼ CUP (59 ML) DRESSING
DRESSING | YIELD: ABOUT 2 CUPS (473 ML)

- -

DRESSING

1 cup (236 ml) low-fat buttermilk

1 cup (245 g) plain fat-free Greek yogurt

¼ cup (59 ml) avocado oil

1 tbsp (15 g) chipotle in adobo, chopped

½ tsp ground cumin

½ tsp garlic powder

1 fresh lime, juiced

¼ cup (13 g) fresh cilantro leaves

2 tsp (10 ml) 100% pure honey

½ tsp black pepper

¼ tsp sea salt (optional)

1 tbsp (15 ml) fresh orange juice

SALAD

6 oz (170 g) grilled chicken breast, chopped small

4 cups (188 g) romaine lettuce, chopped small

½ red bell pepper, seeded, chopped small

1 cup (149 g) cherry tomatoes, quartered

1 bunch scallion, green and white parts, chopped small

½ cup (80 g) red onion, peeled, chopped small

¼ cup (61 g) canned diced green chilies, drained, rinsed

½ avocado, chopped small

2 tbsp (17 g) pumpkin seeds, dry-roasted, unsalted

2 tbsp (14 g) reduced-fat Mexican blend shredded cheese

½ cup (104 g) black beans, canned, drained, rinsed

¼ cup (45 g) sliced canned black olives, drained, rinsed

Place all the dressing ingredients in a blender and blend until combined. Store covered in the refrigerator until ready to use.

In a large bowl, combine all the salad ingredients. If using both servings immediately, add ½ cup (118 ml) dressing and toss to coat. If using only one serving, add ¼ cup (59 ml) dressing to the serving, and toss to coat. Store the remainder of the salad mix and dressing separately, tightly covered, in the refrigerator until ready to use.

- -

NUTRITION (PER SERVING)
Calories 360, Total Fat 16 , Saturated Fat 3.5 g, Trans Fat 0 g, Cholesterol 95 mg, Sodium 340 mg, Total Carbohydrate 20 g, Dietary Fiber 6 g, Sugars 6 g, Protein 36 g, Vitamin A 210%, Vitamin C 120%, Calcium 20%, Iron 15%

- -

ROASTED VEG BUDDHA BOWL WITH TAHINI DRESSING

Wise is the person who chooses roasted veggies with lots of flavor. Well, maybe the Buddha didn't say just that, but your body, mind and spirit will thank you for this one anyway. Pure balance in a bowl!

YIELD: 2 SALADS | SERVINGS: 2 | SERVING SIZE: 1 SALAD + ¼ CUP (59 ML) DRESSING
DRESSING | YIELD: ABOUT 2 CUPS (473 ML)

- -

DRESSING

½ cup (123 g) tahini paste

1 lemon, juiced

1 tbsp (5 g) fresh ginger, grated

1 tbsp (15 ml) 100% pure honey

2 tbsp (6 g) cilantro leaves, chopped

2 tbsp (5 g) basil leaves, chopped

1 cup (237 ml) hot water

SALAD

6 oz (170 g) extra-firm tofu, drained, pressed, cut into 1-inch (3-cm) pieces

2 garlic cloves, peeled, chopped

½ tsp crushed red chili flakes

½ cup (75 g) yellow onion, peeled, cut into 1-inch (3-cm) pieces

½ cup (51 g) celery, cut into 1-inch (3-cm) pieces

¼ cup (31 g) carrots, peeled, cut into 1-inch (3-cm) pieces

½ cup (30 g) cremini or brown button mushrooms, halved

½ cup (50 g) cauliflower florets, cut into 1-inch (3-cm) pieces

½ cup (36 g) broccoli, florets, cut into 1-inch (3-cm) pieces

½ cup (90 g) red bell pepper, seeded, cut into 1-inch (3-cm) pieces

1 cup (70 g) bok choy, cut into 1-inch (3-cm) pieces cubes

½ cup (78 g) frozen shelled edamame, thawed

1 tsp avocado oil

2 tsp (5 g) walnuts, chopped

Place all the dressing ingredients in the blender except the water. While the blender is on slow speed, gradually add the water ¼ cup (59 ml) at a time until well combined. Keep the unused dressing covered tightly in the refrigerator. Shake well as needed before using.

Place the drained tofu on a plate. Top with another plate and then a small can (about 1 pound [454 g]). Allow it to sit for 30 minutes. Remove the can and plate and drain off the excess water. Cut into 1-inch (2.5-cm) cubes.

Preheat the oven to 375°F (190°C). In a large bowl, toss the garlic, red chili flakes, yellow onion, celery, carrots, mushrooms, cauliflower, broccoli, red bell pepper, bok choy, tofu and edamame with the avocado oil to coat thoroughly.

Spread the vegetables evenly over a sheet or cookie tray (2 trays if needed) in 1 layer so as not to overlap.

Roast in the oven for about 15 to 20 minutes or until just tender crisp and starting to brown. Remove from the oven. They can be eaten warm or allowed to cool and be eaten cold.

In a medium bowl, combine all the salad ingredients. If using both servings immediately, add ½ cup (118 ml) dressing and toss to coat. If using only one serving, add ¼ cup (59 ml) dressing to the serving and toss to coat. Store the remainder of the salad mix and dressing separately, tightly covered, in the refrigerator until ready to use.

- -

NUTRITION (PER SERVING)
Calories 310, Total Fat 18 g, Saturated Fat 2 g, Trans Fat 0 g, Cholesterol 0 mg, Sodium 100 mg, Total Carbohydrate 24 g, Dietary Fiber 8 g, Sugars 10 g, Protein 17 g, Vitamin A 120%, Vitamin C 180%, Calcium 25%, Iron 25%

- -

SOUS CHEF SALAD
WITH HONEY-MUSTARD VINAIGRETTE

Every successful chef has a supportive team behind him. Similarly the great ingredients in this salad team up to support your good health moving forward!

YIELD: 2 SALADS | SERVINGS: 2 | SERVING SIZE: 1 SALAD + ¼ CUP (59 ML) DRESSING
DRESSING | YIELD: 2 CUPS (473 ML)

- -

DRESSING

¾ cup (184 g) plain fat-free Greek yogurt

¼ cup (59 ml) Dijon mustard

¼ cup (59 ml) apple cider vinegar

3 tbsp (44 ml) 100% pure honey

1 tbsp (8 g) fresh jalapeño, seeded, minced (optional)

½ tsp ground black pepper

¼ cup (60 ml) extra virgin olive oil

SALAD

6 oz (170 g) cooked lean London broil, sliced thin

2 cups (60 g) baby spinach

2 cups (40 g) arugula

1 cup (180 g) red ripe tomato, chopped

2 slices red onion

2 hard-boiled eggs

½ cup (25 g) scallion, green part only, sliced thin on the bias

½ cup (52 g) cucumber, peel on, sliced thin

2 tbsp (15 g) reduced-fat shredded Swiss cheese

2 tbsp (15 g) reduced-fat shredded mild cheddar cheese

Place all the dressing ingredients except the oil in a blender and blend until combined. With the blender on slow speed, gradually drizzle in the oil until well combined. Store covered in the refrigerator until ready to use.

In a large bowl, combine all the salad ingredients. If using both servings immediately, add ½ cup (118 ml) dressing to the serving and toss to coat. If using only one serving, add ¼ cup (59 ml) dressing and toss to coat. Store the remainder of the salad mix and dressing separately, tightly covered, in the refrigerator until ready to use.

- -

NUTRITION (PER SERVING)
Calories 340, Total Fat 13 g, Saturated Fat 3.5 g, Trans Fat 0 g, Cholesterol 70 mg, Sodium 440 mg, Total Carbohydrate 15 g, Dietary Fiber 3 g, Sugars 10 g, Protein 39 g, Vitamin A 80%, Vitamin C 45%, Calcium 25%, Iron 25%

- -

SEMI-CAESAR SALAD

Some of the calories and fat go bye-bye with this version of the culinary classic. But don't worry, you still get all the flavor.

YIELD: 2 SALADS | SERVINGS: 2 | SERVING SIZE: 1 SALAD + ¼ CUP (59 ML) DRESSING
DRESSING | YIELD: ABOUT 2 CUPS (473 ML)

- -

DRESSING

1 cup (245 g) plain fat-free Greek yogurt

2 tsp (10 ml) Dijon mustard

½ cup (118 ml) red wine vinegar

1 garlic clove, peeled, minced

4 anchovies

½ tsp ground black pepper

Splash cold water, as needed

Dash sea salt (optional)

½ cup (120 ml) extra virgin olive oil

SALAD

4 cups (188 g) chopped romaine lettuce

6 oz (170 g) grilled chicken

1 cup (104 g) cucumber, peel on

1 cup (180 g) tomato, chopped

2 slices red onion, peeled

2 tbsp (10 g) reduced-fat shredded provolone cheese

½ tsp ground black pepper

Place all the dressing ingredients, except oil, in the blender and blend to combine. While the blender is on low speed, gradually drizzle the oil into the blender until emulsified. Keep unused dressing covered tightly in the refrigerator. Shake well as needed before using.

In a large bowl, combine all the salad ingredients. If using both servings immediately, add ½ cup (118 ml) dressing and toss to coat. If using only one serving, add ¼ cup (59 ml) dressing to the serving and toss to coat. Store the remainder of the salad mix and dressing separately, tightly covered, in the refrigerator until ready to use.

- - - - - - - - - - - - - - - -

NUTRITION (PER SERVING)
Calories 300, Total Fat 14 g, Saturated Fat 3 g, Trans Fat 0 g, Cholesterol 95 mg, Sodium 290 mg, Total Carbohydrate 13 g, Dietary Fiber 4 g, Sugars 6 g, Protein 33 g, Vitamin A 180%, Vitamin C 35%, Calcium 15%, Iron 10%

- - - - - - - - - - - - - - - -

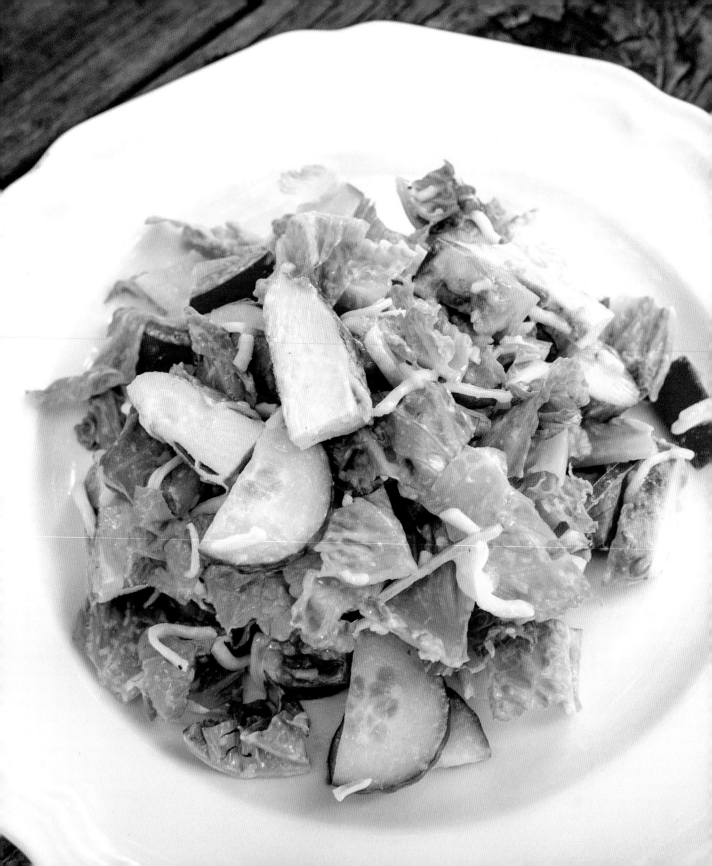

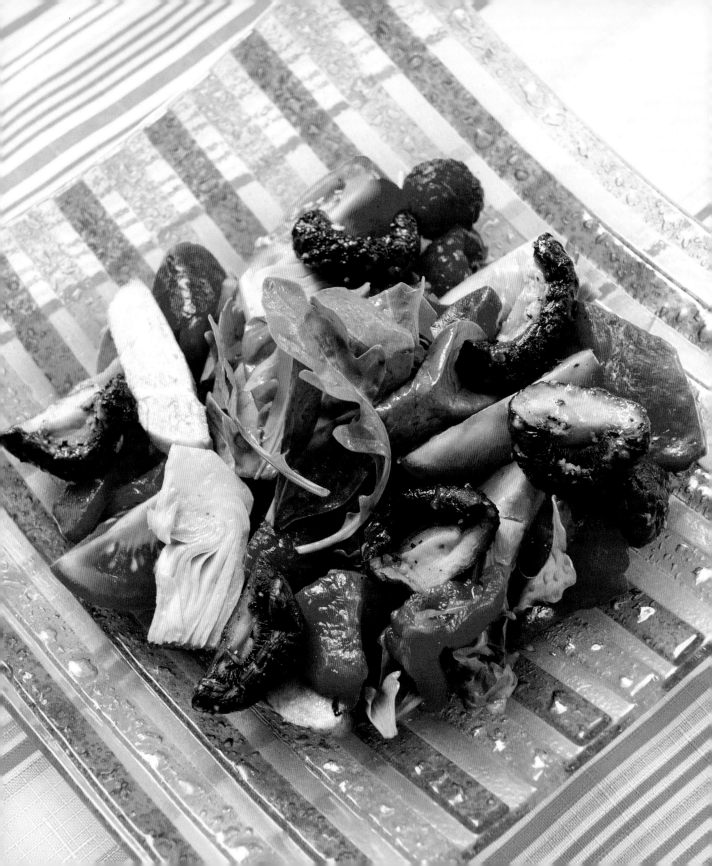

SPINACH-GRILLED CHICKEN SALAD WITH WHITE TRUFFLE SOY VINAIGRETTE

Beware! This is not your average spinach salad with grilled chicken. The otherwise run-of-the-mill combination gets a boost from sweet raspberries, sour lemon, salty soy and a touch of fragrant truffle oil. A combination that transcends the ordinary!

YIELD: 2 SALADS | SERVINGS: 2 | SERVING SIZE: 1 SALAD + ¼ CUP (59 ML) DRESSING
DRESSING | YIELD: ABOUT 1 CUP

DRESSING

¼ cup (59 ml) soy sauce

¼ cup (59 ml) fresh lemon juice

2 tbsp (30 ml) balsamic vinegar

2 tbsp (30 ml) white truffle oil

⅓ cup (78 ml) extra virgin olive oil

SALAD

1 cup (59 g) cremini or brown button mushrooms, halved

1 tsp avocado oil

1 clove garlic, peeled, minced

2 cups (60 g) baby spinach

2 cups (40 g) arugula

6 oz (170 g) grilled chicken

½ cup (84 g) quartered artichoke hearts

½ cup (65 g) roasted red peppers

½ cup (90 g) red ripe tomato, wedges

2 tbsp (15 g) fresh raspberries

1 tbsp (3 g) fresh basil leaves, chopped

Place all the dressing ingredients except for the olive oil in the blender and blend to combine. While the blender is on low speed, gradually drizzle the oil into the blender until emulsified. Keep the unused dressing covered tightly in the refrigerator. Shake well as needed before using.

Preheat the oven to 400°F (204°C). In a medium bowl, toss halved mushrooms with avocado oil and minced garlic. Place on a sheet or cookie tray and bake for about 20 minutes or until softened and starting to brown. Remove from the oven and allow to cool.

In a large bowl, combine all of the salad ingredients. If using both servings immediately, add ½ cup (118 ml) dressing and toss to coat. If using only one serving, add ¼ cup (59 ml) dressing to the serving and toss to coat. Store the remainder of the salad mix and dressing separately, tightly covered, in the refrigerator until ready to use.

NUTRITION (PER SERVING)
Calories 340, Total Fat 18 g, Saturated Fat 3 g, Trans Fat 0 g, Cholesterol 90 mg, Sodium 370 mg, Total Carbohydrate 16 g, Dietary Fiber 7 g, Sugars 6 g, Protein 31 g, Vitamin A 100%, Vitamin C 120%, Calcium 10%, Iron 15%

SUMMER GARDEN SALAD WITH PESTO VINAIGRETTE

A simple and straightforward way to capture the harvest of the summer garden. Crisp, seasonal vegetables star in this easy meal. A fresh herb vinaigrette only enhances the colorful bounty.

YIELD: 2 SALADS | SERVINGS: 2 | SERVING SIZE: 1 SALAD + ¼ CUP (59 ML) DRESSING
DRESSING | YIELD: ABOUT 2 CUPS (473 ML)

- -

DRESSING

1 cup (40 g) Italian parsley leaves, loosely packed

1 cup (24 g) fresh basil leaves, loosely packed

1 tbsp (9 g) grated lemon zest

2 tsp (10 ml) Dijon mustard

¼ cup (59 ml) lemon juice

2 garlic cloves, peeled

½ tsp ground black pepper

¼ tsp sea salt (optional)

½ cup (120 ml) extra virgin olive oil

SALAD

4 cups (400 g) seasonal mixed greens (mesclun mix)

½ cup (55 g) shredded carrots

½ cup (52 g) English cucumber, sliced

½ cup (75 g) cherry tomatoes, halved

2 slices red onion, peeled

½ yellow bell pepper, seeded, thinly sliced

¼ cup (45 g) canned sliced black olives, drained

¼ cup (38 g) reduced-fat feta cheese

2 tsp (7 g) slivered almonds, dry-roasted, unsalted

½ cup (120 g) chickpeas, canned, drained, rinsed

Place all dressing ingredients except the olive oil in the blender and blend to combine. While the blender is on low speed, gradually drizzle the oil into the blender until emulsified. Keep the unused dressing covered tightly in the refrigerator. Shake well as needed before using.

In a large bowl, combine all the salad ingredients. If using both servings immediately, add ½ cup (118 ml) dressing and toss to coat. If using only one serving, add ¼ cup (59 ml) dressing to the serving and toss to coat. Store the remainder of the salad mix and dressing separately, tightly covered, in the refrigerator until ready to use.

- -

NUTRITION (PER SERVING)

Calories 300, Total Fat 21 g, Saturated Fat 4 g, Trans Fat 0 g, Cholesterol 5 mg, Sodium 620 mg, Total Carbohydrate 22 g, Dietary Fiber 4 g, Sugars 5 g, Protein 10 g, Vitamin A 220%, Vitamin C 190%, Calcium 10%, Iron 15%

- -

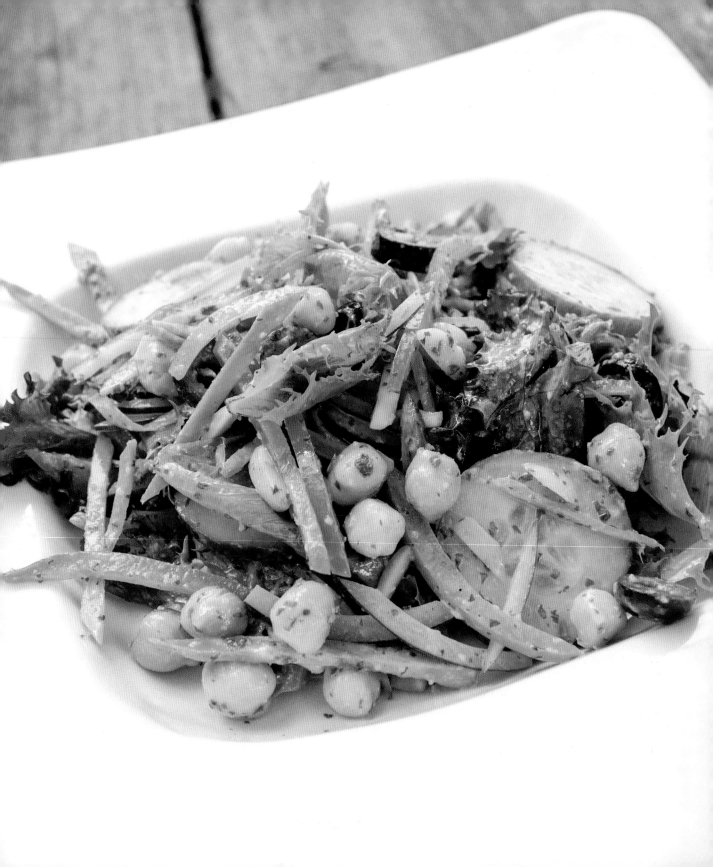

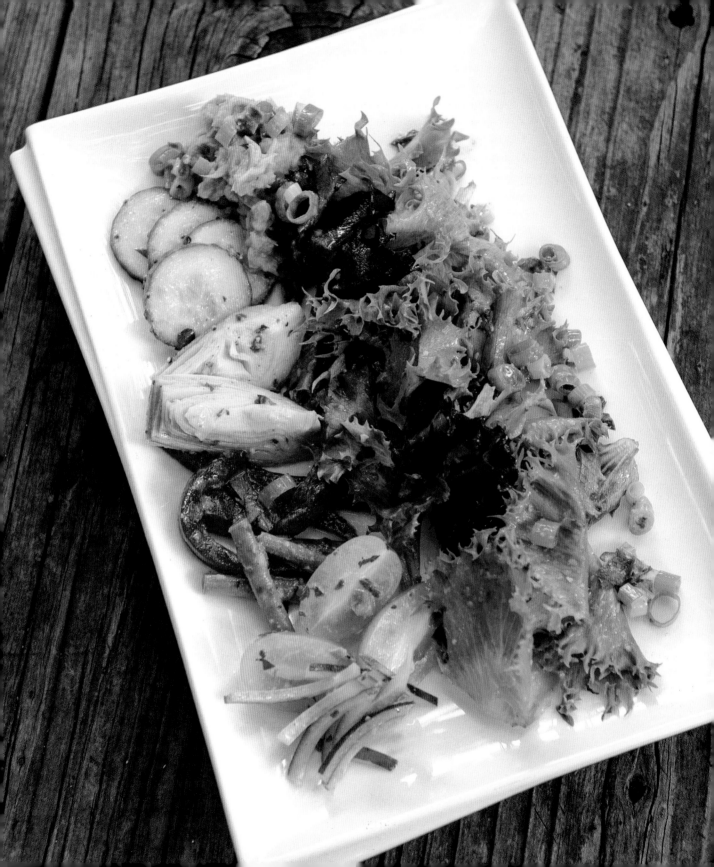

TUNA NIÇOISE WITH CAPER-DIJON VINAIGRETTE

You'll be so busy enjoying the variety and flavors in this salad that you won't have to worry about brushing up on your French to pronounce this salad's name. A satisfied "nice!" will definitely suffice.

YIELD: 2 SALADS | SERVINGS: 2 | SERVING SIZE: 1 SALAD + ¼ CUP (59 ML) DRESSING
DRESSING | YIELD: ABOUT 2 CUPS (473 ML)

- -

DRESSING

½ cup (118 ml) champagne vinegar

2 tbsp (17 g) capers, drained, chopped

6 pitted Niçoise or kalamata olives

2 tbsp (30 ml) Dijon mustard

½ cup (118 ml) cool water

1 tbsp (3 g) Italian parsley leaves

½ tsp ground black pepper

½ cup (120 ml) extra virgin olive oil

SALAD

4 cup (400 g) seasonal mixed greens (mesclun mix)

6 oz (168 g) chunk light tuna

½ cup (65 g) roasted red pepper

½ cup (25 g) scallions, green part only

2 slices red onion, peeled

½ cup (104 g) cucumber, peel on

½ cup (84 g) quartered artichoke hearts, drained rinsed

½ cup (75 g) pear tomatoes, halved

½ cup (55 g) thin green beans, cut into 1-inch (2.5-cm) pieces

2 tsp (7 g) slivered almonds, dry-roasted

Place the dressing ingredients except the olive oil in the blender and quickly pulse blend a few times until combined. While the blender is on low speed, gradually drizzle the oil into the blender until emulsified. Keep the unused dressing covered tightly in the refrigerator. Shake well as needed before using.

In a large bowl, combine all the salad ingredients. If using both servings immediately, add ½ cup (118 ml) dressing and toss to coat. If using only one serving, add ¼ cup (59 ml) dressing to the serving and toss to coat. Store the remainder of the salad mix and dressing separately, tightly covered, in the refrigerator until ready to use.

- -

NUTRITION (PER SERVING)
Calories 320, Total Fat 17 g, Saturated Fat 2.5 g, Trans Fat 0 g, Cholesterol 25 mg, Sodium 300 mg, Total Carbohydrate 17 g, Dietary Fiber 8 g, Sugars 6 g, Protein 25 g, Vitamin A 130%, Vitamin C 110%, Calcium 8%, Iron 20%

- -

TURKEY BURGER TOSTADA
WITH ONE HUNDRED–ISLAND DRESSING

Up your grilled or seared burger game by piling it high with a tower of flavorful salad fixings and topping it off with a tangy special sauce. A burger salad so good you don't need the bun!

YIELD: 2 SALADS | SERVINGS: 2 | SERVING SIZE: 1 SALAD + ¼ CUP (59 ML) DRESSING
DRESSING | YIELD: ABOUT 2 CUPS (473 ML)

- -

DRESSING

1 ½ cups (366 g) plain fat-free Greek yogurt

¼ cup (60 ml) extra virgin olive oil

¼ cup (60 g) ketchup

2 tbsp (30 ml) apple cider vinegar

2 tbsp (20 g) dill pickles, chopped small

2 tbsp (17 g) roasted red peppers, chopped small

¼ tsp ground black pepper

¼ tsp sea salt (optional)

SALAD

2 (4-oz [113-g]) fully cooked (grilled or pan-seared) turkey burgers

4 cups (188 g) romaine lettuce, shredded

4 slices red ripe tomato

2 slices yellow onion, peeled

Place all the dressing ingredients in a small bowl. Whisk together until combined. Keep the unused dressing covered tightly in the refrigerator. Shake well as needed before using.

In a large bowl, combine all the salad ingredients. If using both servings immediately, add ½ cup (118 ml) dressing and toss to coat. If using only one serving, add ¼ cup (59 ml) dressing and toss to coat. Store the remainder of the salad mix and dressing separately, tightly covered, in the refrigerator until ready to use.

- -

NUTRITION (PER SERVING)

Calories 290, Total Fat 16 g, Saturated Fat 3 g, Trans Fat 0 g, Cholesterol 80 mg, Sodium 250 mg, Total Carbohydrate 12 g, Dietary Fiber 3 g, Sugars 7 g, Protein 28 g, Vitamin A 180%, Vitamin C 30%, Calcium 10%, Iron 15%

- -

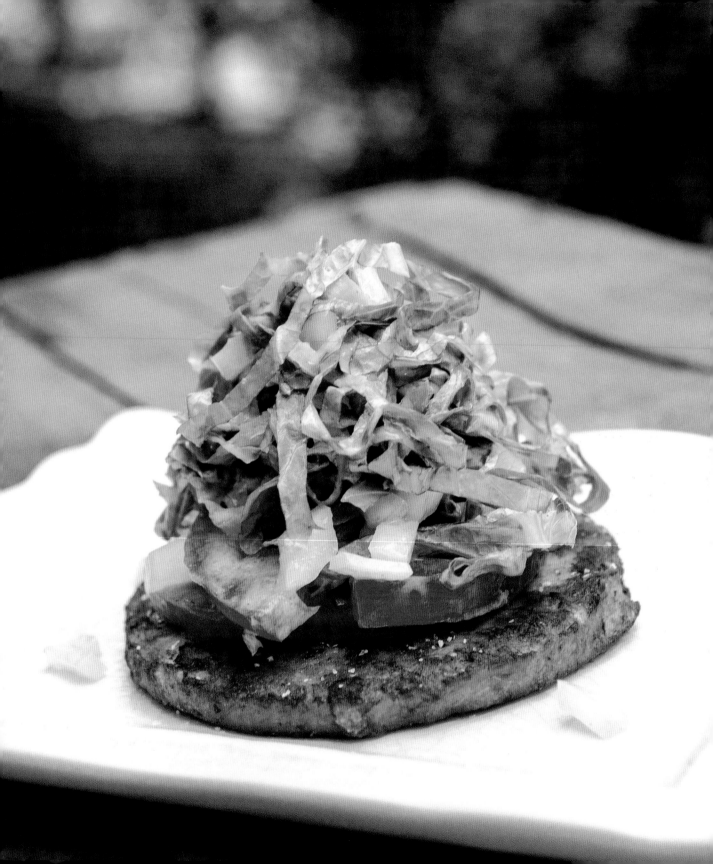

THAI(RIFFIC) SALMON SALAD WITH PEANUT-LIME VINAIGRETTE

Easy, rich canned salmon; fresh, crisp, asian vegetables; and a gingery, nutty vinaigrette provide the foundation for this composed salad. All ingredients that can surely stand on their own, but how good are they together, as a composed salad? The name says it all!

YIELD: 2 SALADS | SERVINGS: 2 | SERVING SIZE: 1 SALAD + ¼ CUP (59 ML) DRESSING
DRESSING | YIELD: ABOUT 2 CUPS (473 ML)

- -

DRESSING

¼ cup (58 ml) fresh lime juice

¼ cup (59 ml) rice vinegar

2 tbsp (30 ml) fish sauce

¼ cup (59 ml) reduced-sodium soy sauce

¼ cup (59 ml) avocado oil

¼ cup (59 ml) water

¼ cup (65 g) all-natural peanut butter

1 tbsp (5 g) fresh ginger, grated

1 garlic clove, peeled, minced

1 tbsp (3 g) fresh cilantro, chopped

1 tbsp (3 g) fresh basil leaves

¼ tsp crushed red chili flakes

SALAD

6 oz (170 g) canned wild salmon, no bones (or precooked salmon)

2 cups (140 g) bok choy, cut thin, on the bias

2 cups (140 g) napa cabbage, shredded

½ yellow bell pepper, seeded, cut thin on the bias

½ cup (52 g) cucumber, peel on, seeded, cut thin on the bias

2 hard-boiled eggs

½ cup (25 g) scallion, green part only

½ cup (55 g) shredded carrots

½ cup (90 g) red ripe tomatoes, chopped

Place the dressing ingredients in the blender and blend to combine and emulsify. Keep the unused dressing covered tightly in the refrigerator. Shake well as needed before using.

In a large bowl, combine all the salad ingredients. If using both servings immediately, add ½ cup (118 ml) dressing and toss to coat. If using only one serving, add ¼ cup (59 ml) dressing and toss to coat. Store the remainder of the salad mix and dressing separately, tightly covered in the refrigerator until ready to use.

- -

NUTRITION (PER SERVING)

Calories 340, Total Fat 16 g, Saturated Fat 2.5 g, Trans Fat 0 g, Cholesterol 50 mg, Sodium 640 mg, Total Carbohydrate 15 g, Dietary Fiber 4 g, Sugars 6 g, Protein 35 g, Vitamin A 230%, Vitamin C 270%, Calcium 25%, Iron 15%

- -

SNACKS

No more pushing through hunger to reach your goals! Snack happy! Keep these simple grab-n-go's ready and available, and stay energized and satisfied throughout the day!

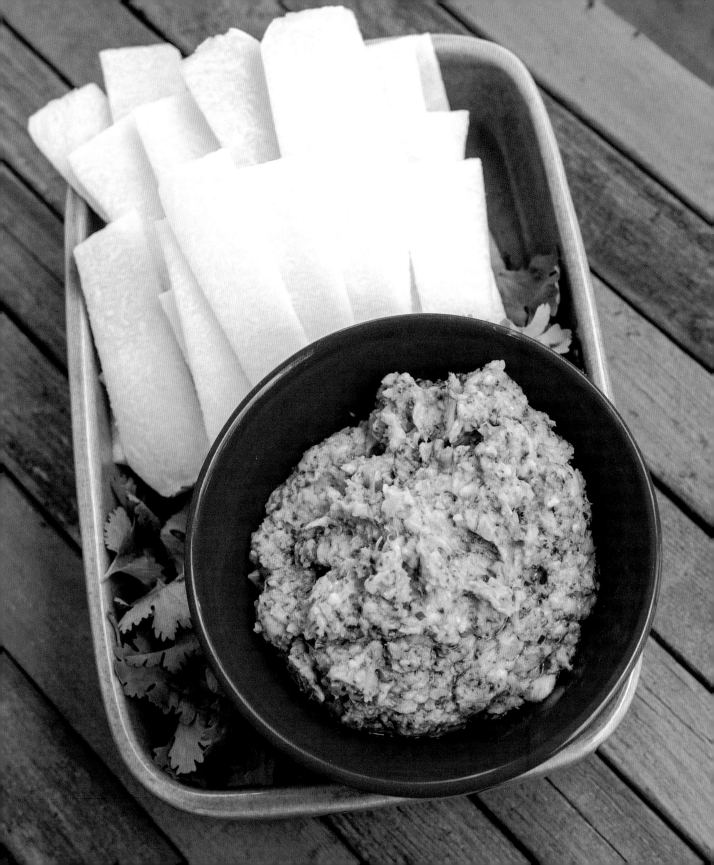

BROCC-AMOLE WITH JICAMA

Nutty roasted broccoli and velvety avocado pair great in this party essential. So deceptively delicious and smooth you'll hardly know you're eating an extra green vegetable!

YIELD: 2 CUPS (473 ML) | SERVINGS: 6 | SERVING SIZE: ⅓ CUP (81 G) DIP + ½ CUP (65 G) JICAMA

2 tsp (10 ml) avocado oil

2 cups (142 g) fresh broccoli florets, cut small

1 medium avocado, peeled, seeded

1 garlic clove, peeled, minced

¼ cup (40 g) red onion, peeled, chopped small

2 tsp (10 ml) lime juice

1 tsp low-sodium soy sauce

1 tsp toasted sesame oil

¼ cup (13 g) fresh cilantro leaves, chopped small

2 tsp (5 g) toasted sesame seeds

½ tsp ground black pepper

3 cups (390 g) jicama, peeled, cut into chips or batons

Preheat the oven to 400°F (204°C). In a medium bowl, mix the avocado oil with the broccoli florets and toss to coat. Spread the broccoli evenly on a baking sheet, and place on the middle rack in the oven.

Bake the broccoli, for about 20 minutes or until it starts to brown and is fork tender. Remove the broccoli from the oven and allow it to cool completely.

When the broccoli is cooled completely, chop it by hand or in a food processor until small.

In a separate medium bowl, combine the avocado, cooled chopped broccoli, garlic, red onion, lime juice, soy sauce, sesame oil, cilantro, toasted sesame seeds and black pepper. Mash the mix until combined.

Serve with jicama or store, tightly covered, (plastic wrap pressed down on top of the dip will keep it from browning) in the refrigerator until ready to use.

NUTRITION (PER SERVING)
Calories 130, Total Fat 9 g, Saturated Fat 1 g, Trans Fat 0 g, Cholesterol 0 mg, Sodium 45 mg, Total Carbohydrate 12 g, Dietary Fiber 7 g, Sugars 2 g, Protein 2 g, Vitamin A 6%, Vitamin C 70%, Calcium 4%, Iron 6%

BUFFALO LEGS

Not a leg man? Try these and you will be! Crispy, juicy, and spicy enough to satisfy any wing lover.
A healthy twist on America's favorite finger food.

YIELD 16 LEGS | SERVINGS 8 | SERVING SIZE 2 LEGS

- -

1 ¼ cups (290 g) low-fat cream cheese, softened

⅓ cup (33 g) scallions, chopped small

2 tbsp (13 g) ground black pepper

2 tbsp (30 ml) red hot sauce

1 tsp fresh lemon juice

¼ cup (28 g) carrot, peeled, grated

¼ cup (45 g) red bell pepper, seeded, chopped small

16 celery stalks, 5-inch (13-cm) long each

In a small bowl, mix together the cream cheese, scallions, black pepper, hot sauce, lemon juice, carrot and red bell pepper. Stir to combine well.

Spread 2 tablespoons (29 g) of cream cheese mix in each piece of celery.

Store tightly covered in the refrigerator until ready to use.

- -

NUTRITION (PER SERVING)
Calories 130, Total Fat 6 g, Saturated Fat 3.5 g, Trans Fat 0 g, Cholesterol 20 mg, Sodium 330 mg, Total Carbohydrate 5 g, Dietary Fiber less than 1 g, Sugars 3 g, Protein 3 g, Vitamin A 25%, Vitamin C 15%, Calcium 8%, Iron 2%

- -

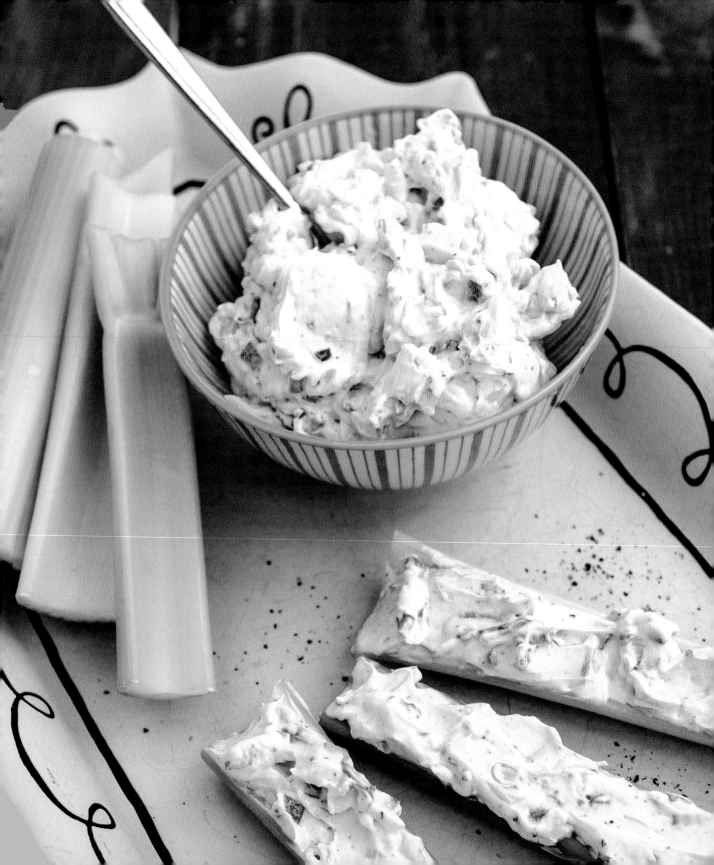

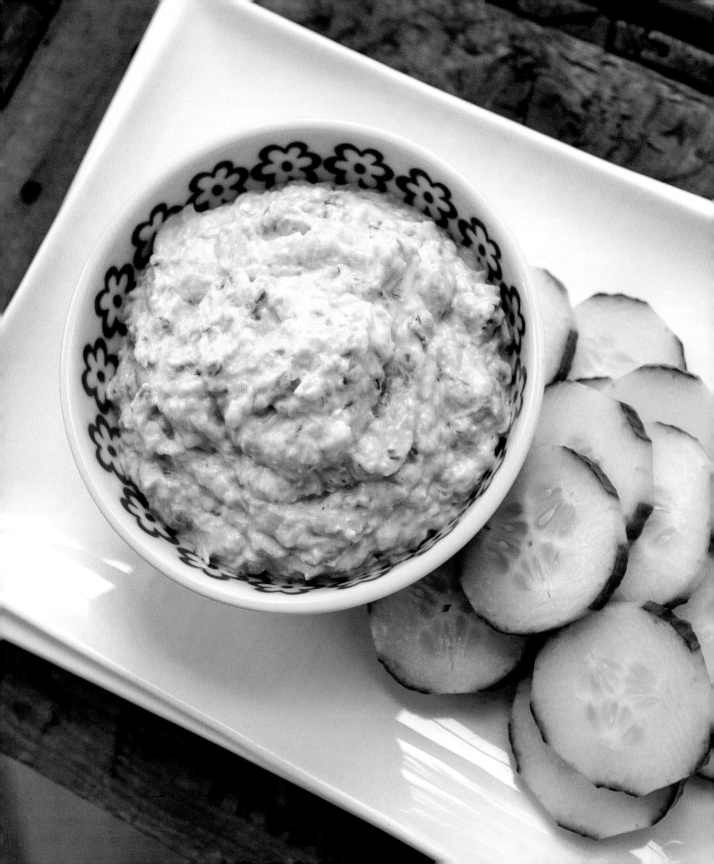

CARAMELIZED 3-ONION DIP

The deep, sweet flavor of caramelized onions, garlic and scallions partner nicely with tangy yogurt to make for a tasty, creamy dip. Make a double batch and keep covered in the fridge. The taste gets better as it sits.

YIELD: 2 CUPS (473 ML) | SERVINGS: 4 | SERVING SIZE: ½ CUP (123 G) DIP + ½ CUP (104 G) CUCUMBER

---

1 tbsp (15 ml) avocado oil

2 cups (300 g) yellow onions, chopped medium

6 garlic cloves

1 cup (50 g) scallion, green and white parts, chopped medium

1 tbsp fresh thyme

½ tsp lemon juice

½ tsp sea salt (optional)

½ tsp ground black pepper

1 cup (245 g) plain fat-free Greek yogurt

2 cups (416 g) English cucumber

Heat the oil in a heavy-bottomed skillet over medium heat. Add the onion, garlic and scallions, and stir to coat. Cook for about 30 minutes, stirring occasionally until the onion mixture is softened and browned. Progressively lower the heat as needed while cooking so as not to burn the onion mixture.

Remove from the heat and fold in the fresh thyme, lemon juice, sea salt (optional) and the black pepper. Stir to combine. Allow it to cool completely.

Transfer the onion mixture to a cutting board or food processor, and chop the mixture small.

In a medium bowl, combine the chopped onion mixture with the Greek yogurt. Cover and allow it to refrigerate for at least an hour before serving with the cucumber.

NUTRITION (PER SERVING)
Calories 100, Total Fat 3.5 g, Saturated Fat 0.5 g, Trans Fat 0 g, Cholesterol less than 5 mg, Sodium 170 mg, Total Carbohydrate 11 g, Dietary Fiber 2 g, Sugars 5 g, Protein 6 g, Vitamin A 4%, Vitamin C 15%, Calcium 8%, Iron 4%

COCOA-MIXED NUT ENERGY BARS

These DIY energy bars are guaranteed to taste way better than any commercial wrapped version. They'll also fend off hunger for a few hours and taste great while doing it!

YIELD: 20 BARS | SERVINGS: 20 | SERVING SIZE: 1 BAR

Cooking spray as needed

¾ cup (60 g) old-fashioned rolled oats

¼ cup (20 g) psyllium husks

¼ cup (43 g) whole raw almonds

¼ cup (32 g) whole raw cashews

¼ cup (31 g) pistachios

¼ cup (38 g) sesame seeds

¼ cup (38 g) chia seeds

¾ cup (194 g) tahini or peanut butter

¼ cup (59 ml) 100% pure honey

¼ cup (22 g) dark unsweetened cocoa

½ tsp vanilla extract

Preheat the oven to 350°F (180°C). Generously coat a 6" × 8" (15 × 20 cm) baking sheet with cooking spray.

In a large bowl, combine the oats, psyllium, almonds, cashews, pistachios, sesame seeds and chia seeds.

Combine the tahini or peanut butter, honey and cocoa in a microwaveable bowl and heat on high for 1 minute. Add the vanilla extract and whisk well until combined. Add the wet mixture to the oat mixture. Stir until well combined.

Pour the mixture onto the prepared baking sheet and with wet hands pat the mixture into a rectangle about 1-inch (3-cm) high. The rectangle will be about 5 × 6-inches (13 × 15 cm). Bake for 15 minutes or until the edges of the rectangle turn golden brown. Do not overbake. The mixture will still feel tacky in the center but will firm up as it cools. When completely cooled, cut into bars.

NUTRITION (PER SERVING)
Calories 140, Total Fat 9 g, Saturated Fat 1 g, Trans Fat 0 g, Cholesterol 0 mg, Sodium 0 mg, Total Carbohydrate 12 g, Dietary Fiber 4 g, Sugars 4 g, Protein 5 g, Vitamin A 0%, Vitamin C 0%, Calcium 4%, Iron 8%

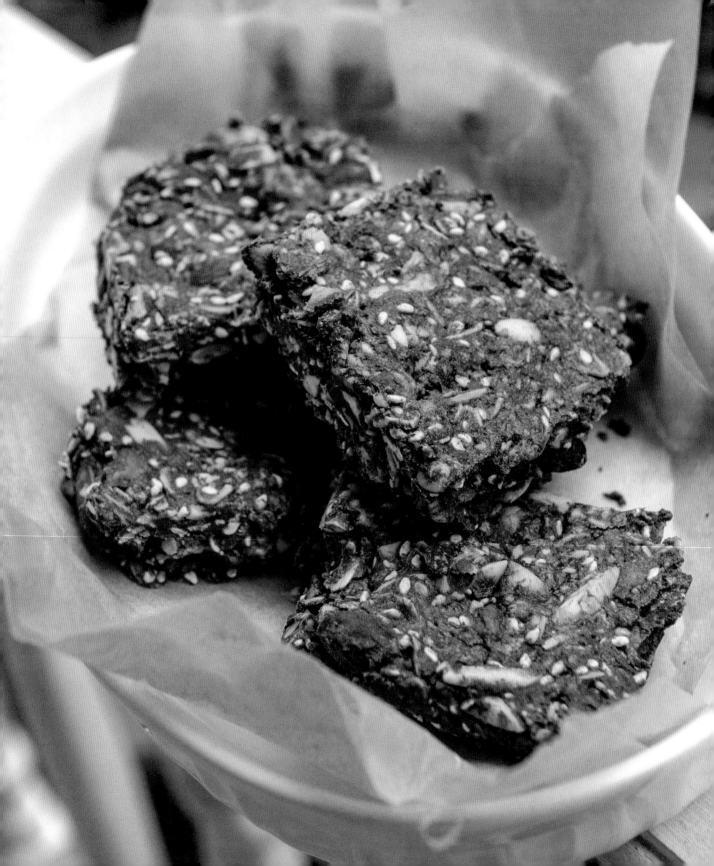

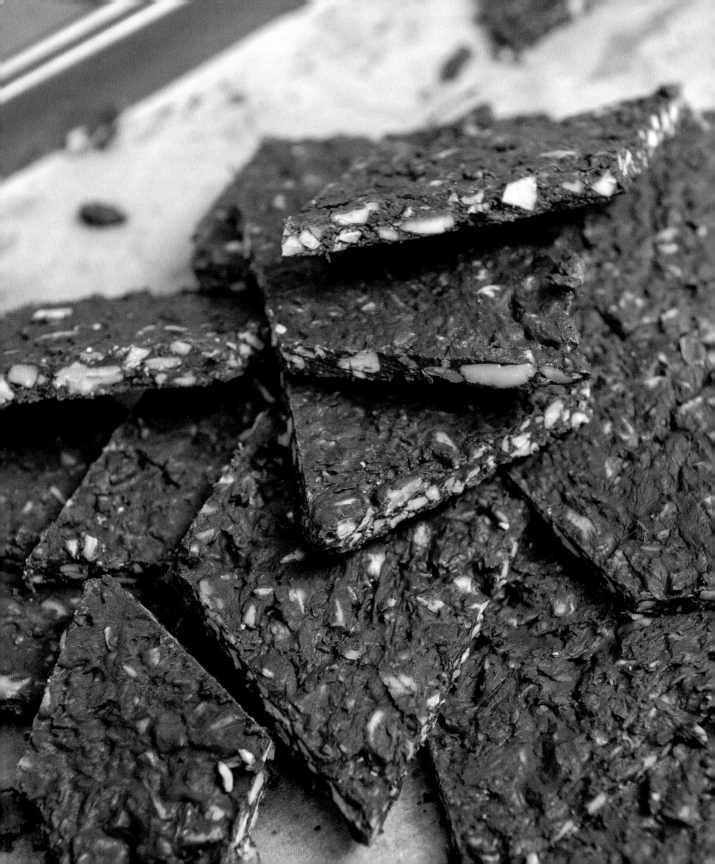

DARK BARK

This bark tastes anything but treelike. Vary the finished product by adding spices like chipotle and ginger, pure extracts like vanilla and orange, even chopped fresh herbs like basil, mint and cilantro. You'll soon agree dark chocolate never tasted so good!

YIELD 3 DOZEN | SERVINGS 36 | SERVING SIZE 1 PIECE

1 ½ cups (180 g) dark chocolate

2 cups (268 g) nuts and seeds (chia, sunflower, hemp, psyllium husk, cashews, peanuts, almonds, walnuts), dry roasted, unsalted, chopped

Line a rimmed baking sheet with foil (avoid wrinkles) or parchment paper.

Melt the chocolate by microwaving on medium for 1 minute. Stir, then continue to microwave stirring every 20 seconds until melted. The chocolate can also be melted in the top of a double boiler over hot (but not boiling) water. Stir the chocolate until melted.

Combine the melted chocolate and the chopped nuts in a medium bowl. Scrape the mixture onto the lined baking sheet and spread evenly into an approximately 12 × 9-inch (30.5 × 23 cm) rectangle.

Place in the refrigerator until it sets.

Transfer the bark and tray lining to a cutting board and use a sharp knife to cut the bark into 1 ½ inch (1.3 cm) pieces

NUTRITION (PER SERVING)
Calories 90, Total Fat 7 g, Saturated Fat 2.5 g, Trans Fat 0 g, Cholesterol 0 mg, Sodium 0 mg, Total Carbohydrate 6 g, Dietary Fiber 2 g, Sugars 3 g, Protein 2 g, Vitamin A 0%, Vitamin C 0%, Calcium 2%, Iron 8%

TIPS: Vary the bark's flavor by adding spices such as chipotle, ginger, sea salt and black pepper.

Use 100% pure extracts like orange, raspberry, vanilla and almond to add flavor too.

Use chopped fresh herbs such as basil, cilantro and mint to add flavor.

Use fresh citrus zest from oranges, limes and lemons to add flavor as well.

DEVILISH EGGS

A less naughty, but equally delicious version of the classic. These assemble in a snap—one bite will make you an "eggspert" on healthy snacking!

YIELD: 8 HALVES | SERVINGS: 4 | SERVING SIZE: 2 HALVES

- -

4 large eggs

½ cup (90 g) small white beans, drained, rinsed

3 tbsp (45 ml) extra virgin olive oil

1 tbsp (3 g) scallion, green part only, chopped small

1 tbsp (15 g) red bell pepper, seeded, chopped small

2 tbsp (22 g) kalamata olives, pitted, chopped small

1 tbsp (3 g) flat-leaf parsley, chopped small

½ tsp Dijon mustard

Smoked paprika, to taste (optional)

Place the eggs in a medium sauce pot. Cover with cold water and bring to a boil. Reduce the heat and simmer for 9 minutes. Drain the hot water and run cold water over the eggs in the pan until cooled completely. Carefully crack and peel the eggs. Cut the eggs in half lengthwise and discard the yolks.

In a small bowl, mash the white beans and olive oil together until smooth. Combine the smashed white bean and olive oil mixture with the scallion, red bell pepper, olives, parsley and Dijon mustard.

Spoon 1 tablespoon (12 g) of the white bean mixture into each of the 8 egg white halves. Sprinkle with smoked paprika (optional) and serve. If not eating immediately, cover tightly and refrigerate until ready to use.

- -

NUTRITION (PER SERVING)
Calories 150, Total Fat 12 g, Saturated Fat 1.5 g, Trans Fat 0 g, Cholesterol 0 mg, Sodium 190 mg, Total Carbohydrate 7 g, Dietary Fiber 3 g, Sugars 0 g, Protein 6 g, Vitamin A 6%, Vitamin C 8%, Calcium 2%, Iron 4%

- -

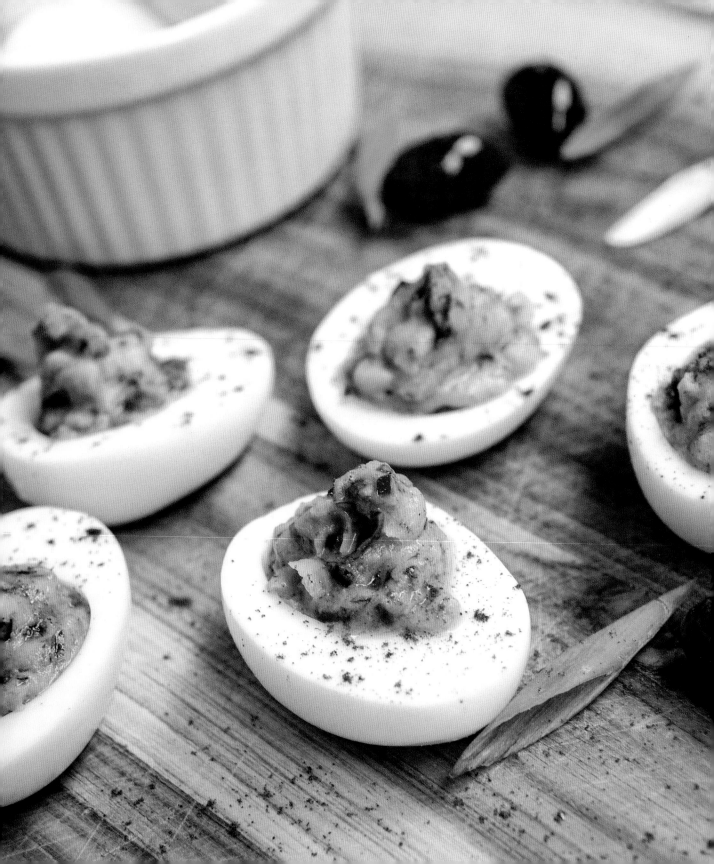

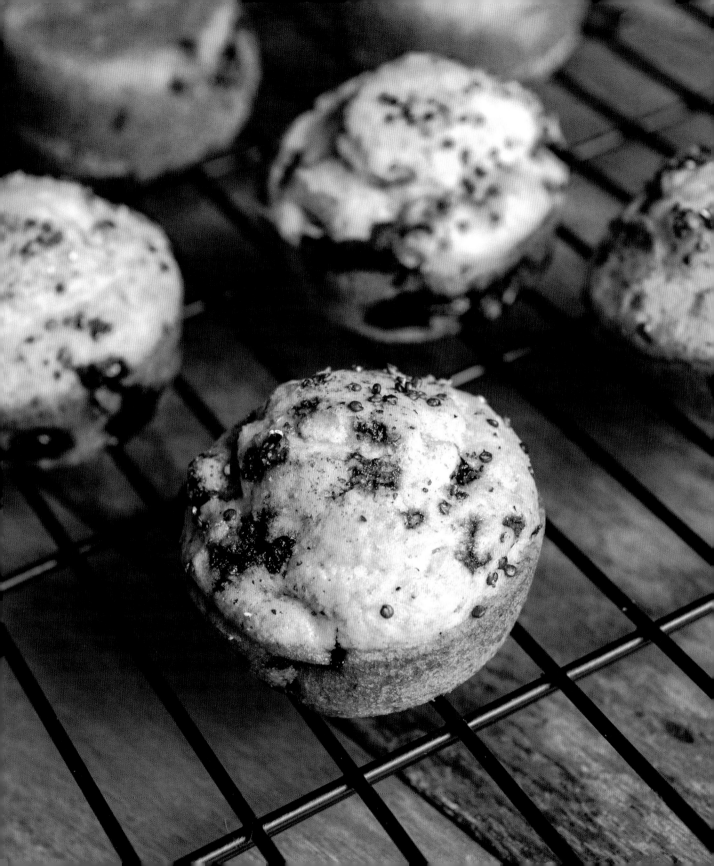

MAN UP BLUEBERRY-ALMOND MUFFINS

Tender, spiced muffins studded with antioxidant-rich blueberries and omega 3-rich chia seeds make for a simple, quick grab-n-go. Vary your berry by using raspberries, blackberries or a combination of all three. Make extra and freeze for the future!

YIELD: 1 DOZEN | SERVINGS: 12 | SERVING SIZE: 1 MUFFIN

---

1 tsp avocado oil

3 cups (289 g) almond meal/flour

½ tsp baking soda

¼ tsp sea salt

1 ½ tsp (7 g) ground cinnamon

½ tsp vanilla extract

½ cup (59 ml) 100% pure honey

6 large egg whites

1 cup (148 g) blueberries,
fresh or frozen

2 tbsp (16 g) chia seeds

1 tbsp (5 g) psyllium husks

Preheat the oven to 325°F (163°C). Lightly oil a muffin pan with the avocado oil. In a medium bowl, combine the almond flour, baking soda, salt and cinnamon.

In a separate bowl, combine the vanilla, honey and egg whites, and gently whisk together.

Add the blueberries to the wet ingredients and stir to combine,

Add the dry ingredients to the wet and mix well to combine.

Divide the batter evenly among the 12 muffin tin holders. Sprinkle the chia seeds and psyllium husks evenly over each muffin.

Bake on the middle rack in the oven for 20 minutes, rotating one quarter turn every 5 minutes. Muffins will be done when the tops start to brown and a wooden pick inserted into the middle comes out clean.

Remove from the oven, and allow to cool for at least 15 minutes before eating. Store unused portions in a tightly covered container.

NUTRITION (PER SERVING)
Calories 190, Total Fat 14 g, Saturated Fat 1 g, Trans Fat 0 g, Cholesterol 0 mg, Sodium 140 mg, Total Carbohydrate 11 g, Dietary Fiber 4 g, Sugars 4 g, Protein 8 g, Vitamin A 0%, Vitamin C 0%, Calcium 6%, Iron 8%

CHEESE AND SNACKERS

A great small plate for a tasty afternoon snack by the fireplace when it's cold or on the deck when it's warm. Good variety and hearty vegetables keeps it satisfying yet nutritious!

YIELD: 1 PLATE | SERVINGS: 1 | SERVING SIZE: 1 PLATE

- -

1 oz (28 g) reduced-fat cheese (sharp cheddar, Swiss, provolone, Monterey Jack, pepper jack), sliced or cubed

1 tbsp (11 g) dry-roasted, unsalted nuts (walnuts, almonds, cashews)

½ cup (84 g) vegetables (artichoke hearts, roasted red peppers, cucumbers, cherry tomatoes, carrots, celery, jicama)

3 kalamata olives, pitted

Arrange on a small plate and serve. If not eating immediately, cover tightly and store refrigerated until ready to use.

- -

NUTRITION (PER SERVING)
Calories 180, Total Fat 12 g, Saturated Fat 3.5 g, Trans Fat 0 g, Cholesterol 15 mg, Sodium 450 mg, Total Carbohydrate 9 g, Dietary Fiber 3 g, Sugars 3 g, Protein 10 g, Vitamin A 4%, Vitamin C 15%, Calcium 30%, Iron 4%

- -

RASPBERRY-ALMOND MOUSSE

This light and creamy no-cook mousse is a cinch to make. Protein-rich tofu, tangy and sweet raspberries and a hint of honey, make this a perfect semi-sweet treat for any season.

YIELD: 6 | SERVINGS: 6 | SERVING SIZE: ½ CUP (202 G)

- -

½ cup (85 g) almonds, whole, unsalted

4 oz (113 g) light soft tofu, drained, patted dry

¼ cup (59 ml) water

2 cups (500 g) frozen raspberries

1 tsp grated lime zest

2 tbsp (30 ml) fresh lime juice

2 tsp (10 ml) 100% pure honey

½ tsp pure almond extract

In a food processor or blender, process the almonds, tofu and water for 3 minutes, scraping the sides as necessary until combined.

Add the remaining ingredients. Process for 4 minutes, scraping the sides as necessary or until almost smooth.

Divide among 4 ½-cup (1-L) glasses and serve immediately, while still cold, or cover the glasses tightly and refrigerate until ready to use.

- -

NUTRITION (PER SERVING)
Calories 130, Total Fat 7 g, Saturated Fat 0.5 g, Trans Fat 0 g, Cholesterol 0 mg, Sodium 0 mg, Total Carbohydrate 13 g, Dietary Fiber 7 g, Sugars 5 g, Protein 5 g, Vitamin A 0%, Vitamin C 35%, Calcium 8%, Iron 8%

- -

ROASTED PEAR WITH CINNAMON RICOTTA AND TOASTED ALMONDS

Supple pears, nutty almonds and smooth ricotta are the perfect trifecta for this clean, simple yet decadent "dessert." The perfect way to end a meal with friends and family.

YIELD: 4 | SERVINGS: 4 | SERVING SIZE: ½ PEAR + 3 TABLESPOONS (47 G) RICOTTA + ¼ TEASPOON CINNAMON + 1 TEASPOON TOASTED ALMONDS

- -

1 tsp ground cinnamon

¾ cup (185 g) part-skim ricotta cheese

2 small Bartlett pears, cored

4 tsp (14 g) dry-roasted slivered almonds

In a small bowl combine the cinnamon and ricotta and set aside until needed.

Preheat the oven to 375°F (190°C). Place the pears on a baking sheet and bake for about 20 minutes or until just fork tender. Remove from the oven.

Top each pear with 3 tablespoons (47 g) of the cinnamon ricotta mix and 1 teaspoon of slivered roasted almonds. If not using immediately, cool completely before storing it, tightly covered, in the refrigerator until ready to use.

- -

NUTRITION (PER SERVING)
Calories 130, Total Fat 5 g, Saturated Fat 2.5 g, Trans Fat 0 g, Cholesterol 15 mg, Sodium 60 mg, Total Carbohydrate 15 g, Dietary Fiber 3 g, Sugars 8 g, Protein 6 g, Vitamin A 4%, Vitamin C 6%, Calcium 15%, Iron 2%

- -

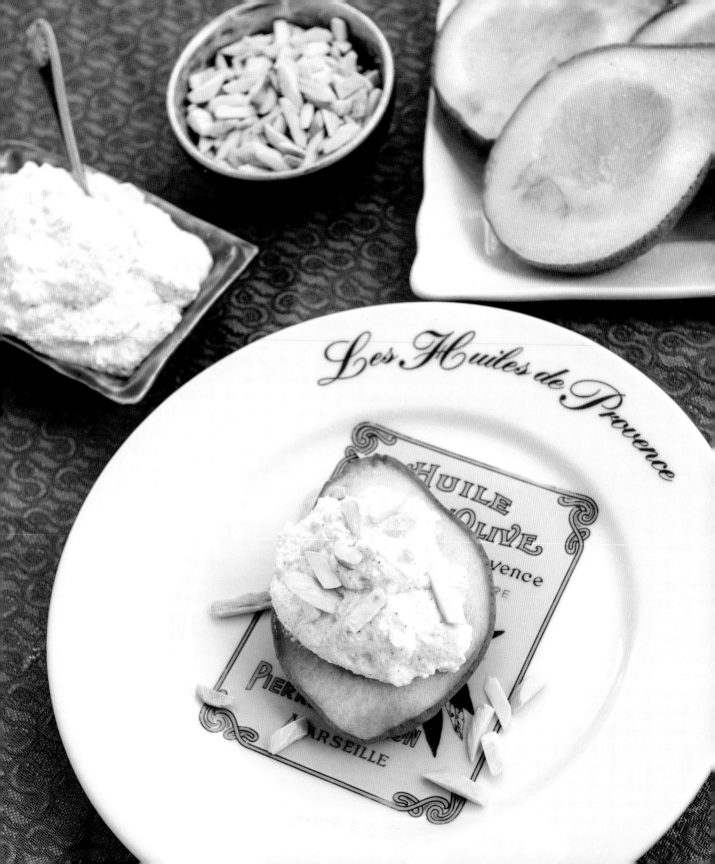

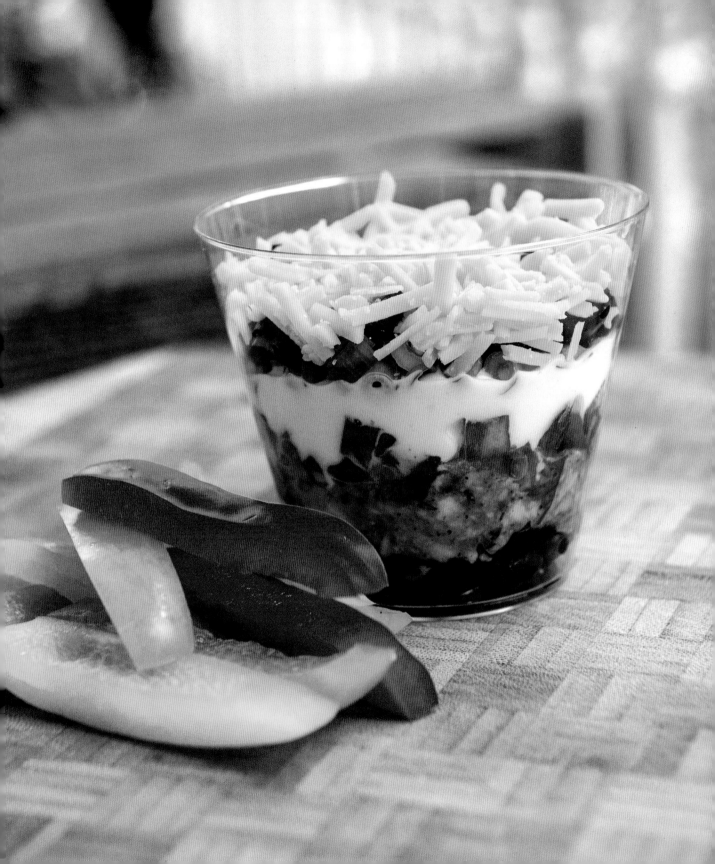

SOUTH OF THE BORDER 7-LAYER PARFAIT

A beautiful, easy-to-assemble, no-cook snack. Make seven of these 7-layer wonders at one time, and have a flavorful go-to item in your fridge for each day of the week.

YIELD: 4 | SERVINGS: 4 | SERVING SIZE: 1 PARFAIT

- -

½ ripe avocado

1 tbsp (15 ml) fresh lime juice

2 tbsp (6 g) fresh cilantro leaves

1 tsp chili powder

½ tsp ground cumin

½ tsp garlic powder

½ tsp onion powder

½ tsp dried oregano leaves

½ cup (104 g) black beans, drained, rinsed

1 cup (180 g) red ripe tomatoes, chopped medium

½ cup (123 g) plain fat-free Greek yogurt

¼ cup (12 g) scallion, green part only, sliced thin

½ cup (90 g) sliced black olives, drained

½ cup (57 g) reduced-fat shredded cheddar cheese

2 cups (350 g) red, yellow and orange bell pepper slices

In a small bowl, mash the avocado, lime juice, cilantro, chili powder, cumin, garlic powder, onion powder and oregano together with a fork.

Into each of four 10-ounce (280-g) containers (plastic cups with lids), place 2 tablespoons (33 g) of black beans, 2 tablespoons (31 g) avocado mash, ¼ cup (45 g) tomatoes, 2 tablespoons (30 g) yogurt, 1 tablespoon (6 g) scallion, 2 tablespoons (22 g) black olives, 2 tablespoons (15 g) cheddar cheese. Cover tightly and store in the refrigerator until ready to use.

Serve with ½ cup (88 g) cut fresh red, yellow and orange bell pepper slices.

- -

NUTRITION (PER SERVING)
Calories 160, Total Fat 8 g, Saturated Fat 2.5 g, Trans Fat 0 g, Cholesterol 10 mg, Sodium 250 mg, Total Carbohydrate 15 g, Dietary Fiber 6 g, Sugars 4 g, Protein 10 g, Vitamin A 45%, Vitamin C 120%, Calcium 20%, Iron 10%

- -

SUMMER BERRY FRO-YO POPS

Creamy frozen yogurt and seasonal berries make these perfect for cooling off on a hot afternoon! Nature's candy on a stick.

YIELD: 8 POPSICLES | SERVINGS: 8 | SERVING SIZE: 1 POPSICLE

- -

2 cups (490 g) plain fat-free Greek yogurt

2 cups (350 g) frozen berries (blueberries, blackberries, raspberries), thawed in the microwave for 1 minute

1 tbsp (15 ml) 100% pure honey

Combine the yogurt, berries, and honey in a blender or food processor. Process until smooth.

Pour into 8 separate ½-cup (118-ml) paper cups or Popsicle molds. Center an unused Popsicle stick in each filled cup.

Freeze until solid and ready to use.

- -

NUTRITION (PER SERVING)

Calories 50, Total Fat 0 g, Saturated Fat 0 g, Trans Fat 0 g, Cholesterol less than 5 mg, Sodium 15 mg, Total Carbohydrate 9 g, Dietary Fiber 2 g, Sugars 4 , Protein 4 g, Vitamin A 0%, Vitamin C 2%, Calcium 6%, Iron 2%

- -

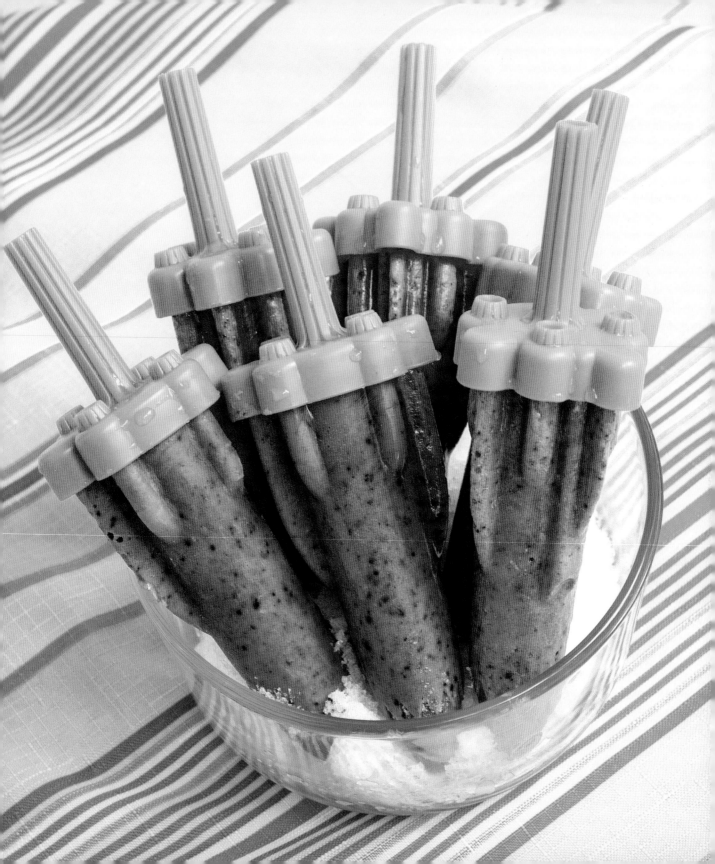

5

HELPFUL HINTS

AND HOW TO KEEP YOUR NEW BODY

During the last seven years I've seen thousands of people like you who were really trying to lose weight and avoid taking medications for their cholesterol and sugar problems. I've used this diet with every single one of them. Not everybody can do it because it is hard in the beginning to imagine life without eating sandwiches for lunch and not having a starch every night on your dinner plate.

In fact, in the diet's first clinical study, over 30 percent of the people couldn't stick to it. But before you despair, one of the most important facts that came out of the first study and was again observed in our larger second study is that over 70 percent of men could keep to this eating plan. For some people, giving up starch is like giving up alcohol or stopping smoking. No longer getting all those nice endorphin (the brain's own heroin) surges any more from eating a piece of cake is something they miss too much. But this eating plan is a man diet, so you'll find this much easier to stick to than your better half might. Another point for our team, gentlemen!

Let's start this section by giving you some helpful hints that I've learned from my many patients along the way. This is spot-on advice that has helped carry them on their journey to slimness and health. I hope these tips will help you too!

MISERY LOVES COMPANY

Some of my most successful patients have found that it is much easier to keep to this dietary regimen when their spouse or even entire family is on the program. People who quit smoking tobacco often do it with a quit buddy, a spouse, friend or acquaintance that is going through the same nicotine withdrawal at exactly the same time as they are. Each buddy can call up and complain to the other one, who can then commiserate and truly empathize. Misery really does love company, and though I don't expect you to be truly miserable with this new way of eating, if you know someone who is doing the program too, you'll have an understanding ear and an empathic shoulder to cry on. There is one caveat, though: pick your buddy wisely. You are looking for a cheerleader or coach to egg you on and help steel your sometimes wavering resolve. Beware a partner who brings you down and demoralizes you instead. Pick someone who is committed to the program, positive about life and easily accessible when you just need to gripe.

If venting your angst publicly is more your particular method of stress reduction, then starting a blog or tweeting can help keep your spirits high and your plate less hazardous. Who knows? If other people around you respond to your messaging, you might even end up creating a little online support group of people going through the same trials and tribulations as you are.

One advantage of declaring your commitment to my diet on Facebook is that nobody likes to publicly admit defeat. You may keep going with it just because you'll be too embarrassed to stop with all your friends and family watching from the sidelines. In fact, there is now a Facebook-like Web site called CalorieKing, where you can post content on a virtual noticeboard, message people and even "friend" them, or not!

In fact, in a study of over 300 people from rural Kentucky, using the power of local community networks (community cooking classes, family fitness fairs and other social activities) allowed participants to lose and maintain their six-pound (2.7-kg) weight loss over a sixteen-month period.

TECHNOLOGY IS YOUR FRIEND

A small digression—bear with me; it will help you, I promise.

In case you are wondering how I know about so many research studies on lifestyle changes, nutrition and so on, I want you to know that I read about four to five studies every day on these topics, to make sure that I am up to date with the medical literature. Therefore, I am going to give you the bottom line of three important technology and weight-loss studies that I have read about recently. But don't worry. Each one will be a single sentence, and all of them will give you great ideas on how to use technology to keep on track.

- Using a health coach (people trained in nutrition and lifestyle change who can help keep you accountable and making good choices) or using self-managed DVDs featuring the Diabetes Prevention Program, together with online tools (the American Heart Association's website for tracking weight and exercise) helped people lose 14 pounds (6.3-kg) and ten pounds (4.5-kg) respectively over a 15-month period. (*Archives of Internal Medicine*, 2012)
- In a randomized trial, adding a personal digital assistant to a standard MD-led weight-loss program led to an almost ten-pound (4.5-kg) weight loss over three months versus only a two-pound (1-kg) weight loss seen with the people on only the standard MD-led program. (*Archives of Internal Medicine*, 2012)
- A review of 14 studies involving more than 2,500 patients by researchers at Columbia University concluded that tracking weight loss on a computer (including online) helps patients shed more pounds than just giving people brochures. But it isn't as good as face-to-face encounters (so feel free to come see me in Connecticut. I accept most insurance plans!). (*Cochrane Review*, 2012)

I recommend to many of my patients that they use their smartphone and download a food-tracking app like MyFitnessPal, livestrong.com's MyPlate or Lose It! that have online communities. These apps are easy to use and they can provide you with such useful information as total daily calories, total carbohydrates (sometimes this can even be broken down into fiber, sugar and starch), total fats and the total amount of protein you are putting in your mouth every day.

If you do use any of these tools, you are aiming for about 1,000 to 1,100 calories per day if you are sedentary (just keep cool—you aren't going to starve, you are still even eating chocolate so how bad can this actually be?). Aim for about 100 grams of total carbohydrates (with about 30 grams of that coming from healthy fiber), around 50–60 grams of fat and 60–90 grams of protein, depending upon your personal preferences.

BE PREPARED

If you were to visit my house at about seven on an average weekday morning, you would be both shocked and amused to see that general chaos and pandemonium abound. I have four kids, three dogs and two hungry cats. Both man and beast must be fed and watered, and everyone wants to enjoy their sacred five minutes of holy bathroom time. The children have to get dressed and the animals are just happy that everyone is awake again and usually decide that this is an opportune moment to play in between our legs! If your life is anything like mine, you'll fully appreciate that there will be no time whatsoever for you to calmly prepare your fresh-cut salad with grilled chicken, low-fat vinaigrette sprinkled with pine nuts and sunflower seeds!

What to do? What to do?

The answer is an obvious one. Prepare all your day's food the night before. Buy a lunch bag and lovingly place into it your lean protein du jour with a salad for lunch, your two fruit snacks, 85 percent dark chocolate and your glorious five o'clock nut bonanza. If you place this veritable feast into the fridge before you go to bed, then it simply won't matter how much havoc abounds in the morning. You will be good to go, literally. To quote my favorite idiom, Food Is Medicine; one should treat food in the same way that people treat their medicine. Many people organize their pillbox the night before so that they don't forget to take their medicine in the mad morning rush. Your lunch box is like their pill box, and it too should be prepared and organized the night before, ready to grab from the fridge at a moment's notice.

TRAVEL SMART

It is one thing to control what you eat when you are at home and are able to limit your food choices, it is quite another thing, unfortunately, when you are out and about, with temptation and peril lurking wherever you turn. There is indeed no place on earth that is more difficult to keep to my eating plan than an airport. Frankly, you would be hard-pressed to keep to any diet while dining at an airport food court, because most everything is junk.

One way to cope with this is to bring your food with you. That is what I always do, and though I have never been questioned about such a practice by the Transportation Security Administration, if I were I would inform them that I am on a strict medical diet and this food is medicine. In the event that you fly with less preparation and forethought, you can purchase nuts and fruit at most places, and if you are willing to sit down and instruct the waiter about the details of your eating plan, he or she will certainly be able to provide you with a lean protein such as fish, chicken, beans or low-fat dairy on a bed of fresh salad.

EATING OUT: WHAT TO ORDER AND WHAT NOT TO EVEN BRING TO THE TABLE

This is a big issue and I want to address it thoroughly because it can become a deal breaker for some people when deciding whether or not to start on the program. But first . . .

There is fascinating study that was published in July 2011 in the *Journal of the American Medical Association* that illustrates the truth behind food labels in restaurants, and the results of this report will definitely help you decide what to and what not to order.

Susan Roberts, PhD and her associates at Tufts University in Boston analyzed 269 meals from a total of 42 restaurants in three states to see if the actual caloric content of each meal was the same as the one advertised on the restaurant's own calorie label. The good news is that overall the labels were pretty accurate. The less than good news is that in the sit-down establishments, the low-calorie options consistently contained more calories than what was stated on the label. This held especially true for carbohydrate-rich food and desserts (which shouldn't surprise you at all, considering they are packed full of starch and saturated fat). Conversely, the foods that were advertised by the restaurants as having the highest calories actually turned out to have less caloric energy than what was written on the label.

Here is my take on the study: Don't rely on the calorie label as a sign that a food is really low-calorie. Just stick to our eating plan of lean protein on a vegetable or salad and you won't be fooled into eating something that is actually much more fattening than you were led to believe.

The other key to eating out successfully is not to allow any starches on your table. Ask the waiter to remove the bread basket, instruct him or her politely that you don't eat rice and not to even bring it to the table. Always enquire about what the accompanying side dish will be so you will not be tempted by a plate of succulent fries glistening with fat right under your nose. It is easier to do this if your dinner partner is on the same eating program. It will take a lot more self-control not to dip into the starchy sides when they are just sitting there in front of you, longingly calling out your name! Don't even put yourself in harm's way.

The same is true for dinner at home with the kids. They may need to eat starch, but you don't. So whatever you do, don't have anything other than veggies or salad on the dining room table, the family starches can be left in the kitchen and can be portioned out there, rather than in the dining room. It will then be much harder for you to get up from the table in front of everyone and do the walk of shame and embarrassment to the kitchen to get your starch fix.

This dietary plan does work when eating out. I do it all the time. My first course is a house salad with an olive oil dressing. This is followed by fish, chicken, turkey or beans on a bed of veggies. When asked, "what side dish would you like with that sir," I always respond the same way, "grilled or roasted vegetables, please, and no potatoes, corn or rice, thank you very much."

Let us briefly discuss fast food so we can have no illusions about a $5 foot-long. In 2013, researchers from Harvard interviewed 1,900 adults, 1,200 teenagers and more than 300 children eating at 89 New England fast-food joints. The results are shocking, and not in a good way. Over one-quarter of everyone interviewed underestimated the number of calories in their meals by over 500 calories! Not surprisingly, the greater the number of calories in the meal, the more likely the person would underestimate the actual caloric content. Both adults and teens who ate at Subway underestimated calorie counts more than any other chain. Just remember—a foot-long sandwich is a lot of starch. So you may be eating a foot-long, but you'll be gaining inches doing it.

SHOPPING HUNGRY, AND READY-MADE MEALS

A study from researchers at Cornell University took 68 adults and told half of them not to eat for five hours before all of them shopped in a virtual supermarket. What they found was that those who fasted were more likely to choose a high-calorie food rather than the lower-calorie alternative compared to the people to had eaten just before shopping. The bottom line is that shopping hungry makes you more likely to make bad food choices.

As I have confessed to you all before, I am not much of a cook; however, you may be more adept in the kitchen than I, so I want to regale you with the results of a study published in the Christmas 2012 edition of the *British Medical Journal.* The study looked at which was a healthier dinner option for the busy person— eating a store-prepared ready-made meal or cooking up a storm at home with the help of a celebrity cookbook recipe. What they found was that the chef recipes had higher calories (not very useful), more saturated fat (not terrible) but less fiber (not helpful) than the store-bought meals. I don't think this will come as a great surprise to some of you: buying a ready-cooked chicken breast with a fresh garden salad from your local store is going to be more nutritious than making a coq au vin.

INTELLIGENT CHEATING

Everybody cheats. You should not be on this diet 100 percent of the time. I would like you to aim to keep true to the plan about 85 to 90 percent of the time. You will still see significant benefits in both your laboratory tests and on your bathroom scale, I promise.

We all know from the outset that you are going to sometimes deviate from this eating plan. Later I'll tell you about a study that discusses the four clinically proven ways that help keep the weight from ever returning. One of those tips is cheating, and you can do it even while you are trying to lose the weight to begin with. However, when you are going to cheat, make it worthwhile.

The study on food labeling in restaurants actually found that the food advertised as the highest in calories was less calorie dense when it was tested in a lab. So pick a top-quality cake or dessert if you are going to have one. Don't waste the calories on something that will be disappointing; spend them on something that will rock your palate and help keep you going until the next indulgence, which won't be for a while!

Remember—eating a dessert once in a while (say one or two times per month) when you just can't take it anymore is fine. But if that becomes a regular occurrence, then dessert will no longer be the exception to the rule; it will be the rule itself. Your weight will stop dropping and even start to rise.

Do you know any marathon runners? Whenever I watch the New York City Marathon, I am struck by how thin and healthy all the runners appear to be. Most of these athletes are eating plenty of starches and clearly have no obvious weight issues.

The reason for this is a simple one. These runners need all the extra calories found in pasta and potatoes that they can get because they are going to be burning them all off as they run, continuously, for many hours.

What can we learn from them?

We can learn that, on the day you cheat, you must burn the excess calories off by doing some extra physical activity. Putting it bluntly, if you want to eat like Michael Phelps, then you need to work out like Michael Phelps too! And if you exercise after a night of indulgence, then you are less likely to look like the Michelin Man and a little more likely to look like Michael Phelps.

DON'T EAT SO FAST, SLOW DOWN

This is probably what your mother always told you, and she was right. It turns out that wolfing down your food will indeed make you fat!

In 2009, Greek researchers investigated the effects on the body of eating ice cream over 5 minutes versus over 30 minutes in some healthy men. What is especially interesting about this particular study is that, as part of the investigation, the scientists decided to measure the levels of some special hormones made in the gut that control appetite.

That's right. Your appetite isn't controlled just by fluctuations in your blood glucose or emotions; it is also controlled by special protein-like substances such as peptide YY (PYY), glucagon-like peptide 1 (GLP-1), ghrelin and leptin that all help let our brain know if we are full or still hungry. Because these substances are important in controlling your appetite, they obviously play a role in weight management. So before we find out the results of our friendly Greek researchers' ice cream trial, permit me to tell you a little more about these hormones.

We shall start off by talking about PYY, GLP-1 and ghrelin, which are all made in different areas of our digestive system.

PYY and GLP-1 are produced by cells in the small and large intestines. They make people feel full by acting on a part of the brain called the hypothalamus, which is thought to control our appetite.

If you are diabetic, you may be familiar with GLP-1 because of one of the other effects it has on your body: making your pancreas release more insulin into the bloodstream to help keep your sugar levels under control. Incidentally, some of the flashiest new diabetic drugs on the market, like Byetta and Victoza are basically just synthetic versions of GLP-1, and these drugs not only lower your blood glucose, but they also help you lose weight, perhaps due to the effect they have on your appetite.

Ghrelin is made in the cells of your stomach and pancreas. That rumbling, grumbling feeling you sometimes get in your stomach when you are hungry is caused by the release of ghrelin, which also tells parts of your brain that you are hungry.

Just before we return to our Greek friends and learn what they found out after feeding people ice cream, let's look at one more substance that is also very important to how our body signals our brains to let us know whether we are hungry or full.

Researchers have known about the hormone leptin (which comes from the Greek word *leptos*, meaning "thin") since the 1950s. The original research was done on mice that were superfat and very hungry all the time. It turned out that they had a leptin deficiency. When they were given leptin injections, they all slimmed down to a normal size—for a mouse.

Now whether this can be translated into a weight-loss drug for humans is still unknown, since mice are mice and humans are humans, but there can be no doubt that leptin influences our appetite, and drug companies are currently studying synthetic versions of leptin to help treat diabetes and obesity.

And now back to Greece.

Seventeen healthy young men were given almost 700 calories of ice cream to eat within five minutes. The researchers took blood samples from the subjects before and after their binge and measured levels of PYY and GLP-1 (which make you feel full) and ghrelin (which makes you feel hungry).

The researchers did the experiment again, but this time, they let the men enjoy the sweet, cool snack over a more relaxed half hour, again measuring the levels of those substances in their bloodstream before and after the snack.

They found that the GLP-1 and PYY levels were significantly higher when the men ate slowly, compared to when they wolfed down the ice cream in five minutes flat! Translating this into plain English, if you eat slower you feel fuller due to higher GLP-1 and PYY levels than if you bolt food down as fast as you can.

Interestingly, the ghrelin levels in the bloodstream, which tell you that you are hungry, did not change whether the men ate quickly or slowly.

Based on this study, it seems that eating slowly makes you more satiated, compared to eating food at a fast and furious pace. Since feeling full makes you less likely to want to eat more, it appears that your mother's old saying is true: wolfing down your food will make you fat. Good for you, Mom!

WHAT'S THE DEAL ABOUT EXERCISE?

There is no way I could write about how to naturally lose weight, drop your sugar levels and lower your cholesterol without talking about exercise. In my first published clinical trial, over 60 percent of the successful and motivated participants were already doing at least 150 minutes of exercise per week before they were even on the eating plan. Despite that high level of exercise, their baseline lab tests were still high, and it was clearly the diet that made their numbers nose-dive not just the daily sweat in the gym. However, you should not have any doubt about the incontrovertible scientific fact that exercise will literally save your life. As one of my patients told me, "Sitting is the new smoking."

I want to begin this section by talking about what type of exercise is most useful in battling metabolic syndrome. We shall then review the most recent research that shows us what exercise can and can't do for you in terms of weight loss. Finally, we'll look at the science behind whether intense exercise like ultramarathon running or iron man competitions is really good for your body or not.

One of my pet peeves is directed to many of my esteemed and well-intentioned medical colleagues. When you go to your doctor's office and he or she starts you on a new medication, the doctor always gives you specific instructions: the name of the drug, how much to take and when to take it. If food is medicine, exercise is too! So telling a patient simply to get more exercise without giving specific instructions is like prescribing a new medication without giving the patient the name, dose or even how frequently he or she should be taking the thing!

Luckily for all of us, there is a well-known tool that can help us write an exercise prescription. It is called a FITT prescription, which stands for frequency, intensity, type and time. Let me give you an example.

If I were to write you a FITT prescription on my prescription pad, it might look something like this:

- Frequency: Two to three times per week
- Intensity: Heart Rate (HR) 120 beats per minute (bpm) or according to the perceived exertion scale
- Type: Speed walking
- Time: 20 minutes

You see how you now know exactly what to do?

Your medicine isn't Lipitor 10 mg every night; it is speed walking for twenty minutes, twice a week and getting your heart rate up to around 120 bpm while you are on the trot!

Let's go over the rules for a FITT prescription in more detail so, if your doctor doesn't prescribe it, you can design your own one and customize it to your liking.

FREQUENCY

Exercising two to three times per week is an ideal beginning. If you do something on both Saturday and Sunday, you have only one more session to do during the rest of the work week. It would obviously be preferable if you could exercise every other day, rather than saving it all up for the weekend, but whatever you do that works within the confines of your busy schedule is a great start.

As far as what an ideal frequency would be for all you over achievers out there, the Institute of Medicine recommends 60 minutes of moderate-intensity physical activity every day. The American College of Sports Medicine is a little more moderate with its recommendation of 30 minutes of moderate-intensity activity on a daily basis. Either way, the eventual goal is to move daily. That was how the body was designed to operate when we were all hunter-gatherers, and that is what you should aim to do in due course—minus the stone spear!

INTENSITY

A typical prescription would read, "Heart Rate 120 bpm or measure the intensity by using the perceived exertion scale." We are aiming for an aerobic level of exercise. There are two simple ways for you to tell if you are hitting that or not. One is the well-oiled technique of monitoring your heart rate during the activity. You want to be at 70–80 percent of your maximum heart rate for most of the time. The easiest way to work out your maximum heart rate is to use the following calculation:

220 - Your Age (in years) = Your Maximal Heart Rate

Though I can't believe it, I am 44 years old with some specks of gray fairy dust on the sides of my head. My maximal heart rate, therefore, is 220 minus 44, which is 176 bpm.

Based on this calculation, for me to be in an aerobic zone during my elliptical or bike "hit," my heart rate needs to range between 124 bpm (which is 70 percent of my maximal 176) and 142 bpm (which is 80 percent of my maximal 176).

The good news is that most of today's aerobic equipment such as treadmills, elliptical machines and exercise bikes can monitor your heart rate while you are exercising so you know whether you need to push harder or pull back a little to stay in that 70–80 percent range.

If math is not your thing or you don't have access to an exercise machine, then you can go old-school or classic, and walk like our ancestors did. To determine how fast you need to walk to get to an aerobic level of activity, you can use the perceived exertion scale. You see, it turns out that if you are at an aerobic level of activity, you won't be able to hold a conversation. You may be able to say a few words, but anything more than that will be difficult.

Now back to the science before we talk about the veritable smorgasbord of exercise options for you to try.

Question:

If you are in a time crunch, what is the best bang for your buck in terms of exercise intensity? Is it hard and fast or slow and steady? Luckily for us, we have two Scandinavian studies that answer this very question.

Study numero uno looked at 10,000 Danes and found that a brisk walk halved the risk of developing metabolic syndrome over the ten-year study. In contrast, a leisurely stroll for even more than one hour per day had no preventive effect.

Study numero dos from Norway followed healthy but inactive and overweight 35- to 45-year-old men during a ten-week exercise regimen. They found that only 15 minutes of high-intensity exercise three times per week led to significant health benefits.

But before you all start killing yourself with 15-minute bursts of exercise insanity, permit me to make one very important point.

There are no prizes for being an idiot. If you haven't done any exercise for years and are out of shape, please see your doctor before you begin your new exercise revolution. I have seen three male patients over the last few years who had heart attacks while they were in the gym overdoing it.

Knowing your maximal heart rate is not some kind of personal challenge for you to see if you can reach it. If you try to hit the maximal speed of your car, you might burn out the engine. Let's not try the same thing with your heart, shall we.

TYPE

The type of exercise—speed walking, for example—is part of the prescription. Let's briefly review two important studies that will help us figure out whether we need weight training, aerobics or a combination of both to keep us in good shape and help us reverse our metabolic syndrome.

In September 2011, a research team from Duke University published the results of their study, Studies of a Targeted Risk Reduction Intervention through Defined Exercise (STRRIDE) in the *American Journal of Cardiology*. The investigators recruited 196 overweight and sedentary men and women aged between 18 and 70 and randomly divided them into three groups. The first group did three sets of exercises on eight different weight machines three times per week, the second group did 120 minutes per week of aerobic activity on an elliptical bike or treadmill, and the final group did both. Every participant had to stay on the program for eight months, long enough to see if there were any big changes in terms of their metabolic syndrome.

It comes as no surprise that, although the people in the group that did weights and aerobics adhered less to the program compared to the participants in the other two groups, their waist circumference, triglycerides and other features of metabolic syndrome improved the most.

What is interesting is that the aerobics-only group also saw improvement in their metabolic syndrome, but the weight training-only group did not see any change in their metabolic syndrome, although they did become more fit.

The researchers concluded that "aerobic training alone was the most efficient mode of exercise for improving cardiometabolic health."

So aerobic activity is definitely required, but are there really no metabolic benefits to weight training? Let's look at another study and decide this one for ourselves.

In July 2011, Dr. Preethi Srikanthan and colleagues from UCLA published a new analysis of over 13,000 participants from the NHANES III survey, a survey with which you are familiar.

They looked at the amount of muscle, or muscle mass, that each participant had, and then correlated that to their risk of developing diabetes. What they found was quite remarkable. Those people with the highest body muscle mass had 63 percent less chance of getting diabetes compared to those with the least amount of muscle on their bodies. In other words, the more your body is composed of muscle rather than fat, the less chance you have of developing diabetes or sugar issues. So having muscle is a good thing and therefore weight training to increase lean muscle mass is a good thing too!

In the last analysis, in terms of the type of exercise you should do, the best results come from a combined approach of aerobics and weights. If you have a gym membership and are unsure how to use those machines, which sometimes resemble medieval torture devices, get yourself a personal training session or two and let a professional show you how to kick your own butt.

TIME

Your exercise goal should be 20 minutes. But start with five minutes and go up. This isn't a race, and you can work up slowly till you reach the American College of Sports Medicine's 20–30 minutes of exercise per day. Working your way up to the Institute of Medicine's hour of exercise per day would be awesome, but as I don't have enough time in my day for that, I wouldn't ask you to do anything that I don't do myself.

And yes, dear reader. I also keep to my own diet, and I am happy to report that my weight is good and my cholesterol is 140 without the help of medicine, just food!

Two more interesting facts and we shall be done with exercise. The first is rather a depressing one. According to scientific studies, exercise is more a weight maintenance tool rather than the weight-loss pill many people had hoped for.

In 2010, researchers at Harvard reported the results of an analysis they had done on data from over 34,000 women in the Women's Health Study, which had run for fifteen years. They found that a woman of normal weight has to walk for 60 minutes or jog for 30 minutes every day just to maintain her weight. If she works out less than that, she is much more likely to put on weight over a three-year period.

Now for the really bad news.

Exercise has no effect at all on weight control for an overweight woman (with a body mass index greater than 25). In other words, walking one hour a day or jogging for 30 minutes every day is still not sufficient for an overweight woman to control her weight, let alone lose some.

Again, exercise is critical; humans were designed to move every day. You are human, so you were designed that way too! Exercise reduces your risk of cancer, heart disease, diabetes and depression to name just a few of its many, many health benefits.

The most recent scientific studies suggest that exercise alone is not an effective weight-loss plan. Exercise helps you keep your weight stable; but if you want to lower it, you must restrict your calories, plain and simple.

Can you overdo exercise? Can you cause yourself damage by overexercising? The answer appears to be yes. But you have to really overdo it!

In this Australian study that was published in the December 2011 issue of the *European Heart Journal*, 40 competitive endurance athletes (marathon runners, triathletes, alpine cyclists and so on) were examined before and after their various races. Just so you know how hardcore these folks were, they all trained hard, at least ten hours every week, and all finished within the top 25 percent of every race.

These, my friends, are the people who live to exercise and may be addicted to the endorphins they get from putting their body through hours of extreme exertion.

The researchers put all these athletes into an MRI machine and looked at what happened to their heart function before and after their races.

What they found was remarkable and not completely surprising. The right side of their heart (which is responsible for pumping blood to the lungs) functioned much worse immediately after the race and then eventually returned back to normal. They also found that the levels of special enzymes in the blood that indicate damage to the heart muscle were increased straight after the race. In fact, in an accompanying editorial to the study, two noted British cardiologists even raised the possibility that "repetitive bouts of arduous exercise" may result in significant damage to the right heart muscle.

Please do not take away from this cautionary study that I don't think we all need to exercise. We do. I am just not sure that we need to regularly put our bodies through hours upon hours of strain and sweating. That might simply be too much of a good thing.

THE BETTER YOU SLEEP THE THINNER YOU WILL BE

There are three things humans need to be able to do well just to stay healthy. They are all obvious, and most people are pretty lousy at doing any of them, which is why we are all so unhealthy.

We need to eat properly, which I hope you are now doing with a little help from this book. We also need to move every day because our bodies are designed for hunting and gathering, which demands a fair amount of daily physical activity if you want to eat rather than starve. The third piece of this trifecta involves sleep.

If you want to get a big tick in the column titled Sleep, you need to be able to go to sleep when you are tired, fall asleep easily, sleep through the night and wake up refreshed in the morning without an alarm. And you need to do all of that without the help of any kind of sleeping pill!

The point of sleep, my friends, is to wake up refreshed. I don't mean that you all have to be giddy happy and irritatingly chirpy at 6 a.m., just refreshed. To help you along the way to a peaceful night, you might like to remember the following tips:

In the same way that some women need to be in the mood for love and intimacy, your body needs to be in the mood for sleep. So set the scene so you can seduce your body into slumber.

The temperature in your bedroom should be to your liking, the noise level low, the lights should be dimmed so that the body's natural sleeping aid, the hormone melatonin, can flow freely and in abundance and help signal the body that bedtime is finally here. Your bed should be comfortable, your pillow too. The TV should be off so that it is not stimulating you and keeping you awake.

Stop drinking any caffeinated drinks from the early afternoon onward, so that your body isn't fighting the stimulating effects of the caffeine still in its bloodstream at ten o'clock at night. And empty your bladder before you lay down for the night. If you have a tendency to wake up during the night to urinate, not drinking after dinner may help keep your bladder less full and your sleep less fractured.

What has sleep got to do with weight loss, you might be thinking. A lot, is the answer.

In March 2011, the results of a six-month trial in which more than 470 overweight men and women participated were published in the *International Journal of Obesity*. All the participants went on an intensive weight-loss program that included a calorically reduced (by 500 calories) diet high in fruits and veggies and low in saturated fats, three hours of exercise per week and a number of group sessions where daily diet diaries were reviewed and any problems were discussed and solved. The cool thing about this government-funded study is that the stress levels and average time these individuals spent asleep was also recorded.

The unsurprising news is that the average person lost 14 pounds (6.3-kg) over six months on this program. Not bad, though I do find that those taking my dietary approach tend to lose more than that after six months. However, the reason I am telling you about yet another weight-loss trial is because of what the researchers also discovered.

When these scientists analyzed the data from this study, they found that the degree of success people had on the program could be predicted by their stress level and the amount of time they slept at night. Success in losing ten pounds (4.5-kg) (which was the goal of the trial) was much more likely if people slept between six and eight hours per night. People who slept fewer than six hours were much less likely to hit that magic ten pound (4.5-kg) number.

Not surprisingly, the researchers also found that people who had the least amount of stress had the best chance of losing weight. Stress is something we learned about when we discussed cortisol, the body's stress hormone, high levels of which can definitely sabotage weight loss.

So now you can see why sleep is so important to our little adventure together. And by the way, though nobody knows for sure, the latest research suggests that our newest friends, ghrelin and leptin, the neuropeptides that control our appetite, may be to blame for the fact that poor sleepers can't lose weight.

One more brief study on the benefits of sleep before we move onward and upward. In July 2013, Dutch researchers published the results of a 15,000-person study that looked at lifestyle changes and the risk of dying of a heart attack. The results were hardly earth-shattering. If you do four things, exercise, keep to a healthy diet, limit your alcohol intake and don't smoke, your risk of dying of a heart attack plummets by a nice 67 percent. The cool part of the study is that the researchers also looked at how long everybody slept. Here is what they found: the risk of dying of a heart attack for those who slept more than seven hours every night and did the other four things dropped by a total of 83 percent. Clearly, then, when it comes to the trifecta of good health—eating well, moving often and sleeping soundly—the sum is greater than its parts.

CHEMICALS THAT RAISE YOUR CHOLESTEROL AND INSULIN LEVELS AND MAKE YOU FAT

Not only what you cook but also what you cook *in* has an effect on your cholesterol. There is new research showing that kids who eat food cooked in nonstick pots and pans have an increase in their bad cholesterol. This is due to the perfluorooctanoic acid (PFOA) and perfluorooctane sulfonate (PFOS) that are found in such pots and pans, and we'll now talk about what they are and why you don't want to eat then. Let's start by giving you the low-down on PFOA and PFOS, the chemicals that are used in the manufacture of cookware to make our pots and pans become of the nonstick variety.

Scientists have known for a while that when adults are exposed to PFOA and PFO, their LDL levels go up. To investigate whether this also happens in kids, researchers from West Virginia University analyzed blood samples from 12,476 kids in the Ohio and West Virginia area who had all been exposed to PFOA and PFOS from contaminated drinking water.

They found that the higher the children's blood levels of PFOS and PFOA, the higher their total and LDL cholesterol readings were. They also saw that the high levels of PFOS were associated with a decrease in HDL, the good cholesterol. This is chilling stuff, don't you think?

It appears that everybody is exposed to these chemicals and they have even been found in food packaging, breast milk and in the air we breathe!

Now I don't recommend we stop breast feeding our young or breathing air, but I do think this is a cautionary tale, and we should be aware that our environment can be polluted and all these chemicals can have significant effects on us and our children.

Here are two more chemicals that you want to avoid: bisphenol A (BPA) and di-2-ethylhexyl phthalate (DEHP)—I would love to meet the genius who came up with that name!

BPA, which is found in plastic water bottles and other types of food packaging, has been shown by researchers at the University of Michigan to be associated with an increased risk of obesity in kids. And since most of us were once kids, we should probably steer clear of BPAs also, so use metal or BPA-free water bottles to hold your daily 64 ounces (2 L) of cool, clear, H_2O.

Urinary levels in adolescents of di-2-ethylhexyl phthalate (DEHP), the other chemical to avoid, which is also found in plastic, was measured by researchers at NYU. They found that for every threefold increase in the concentration of DEHP in the urine, there was a 27 percent increased risk of the kids developing insulin resistance. Again illustrating the point that it isn't just what you eat, but also what you eat it in that counts.

GUT FLORA, ANTIBIOTICS AND THE MIDDLE-AGE SPREAD— THERE IS A CONNECTION

Did you know that over the last 50 years Americans have grown one inch (2.5 cm) taller and 24 pounds (10.9-kg) heavier than they were in the 1960s? Why is that? Better nutrition? More exercise?

There may be many reasons, but a fascinating article published in the March 8, 2014, edition of the *New York Times* suggests that the reason may actually be overuse of antibiotics in animal feeds, causing our native gut flora to be altered and making us fat.

We have billions of bacteria that colonize our gut right after birth. These microscopic friends are essential to our health. In fact, the latest research suggests these friendly bacteria are connected, not just to good bowel health, but also to the risk of developing heart disease and even cancer. Remember, they live inside us, so if we die, they do to!

The *Times* article describes a study by researchers at NYU that aptly illustrates the connection between antibiotics, gut flora and weight gain. In the study, scientists took two groups of baby mice and gave all those big-eared rodents lots of high-calorie food. In addition, they administered an antibiotic to the mice in one of the groups. What they found was frightening.

The mice that were given the antibiotics put on twice as much weight as the other mice. Now remembering that all the mice got the same number of daily calories, the researchers concluded that it was the addition of the antibiotic that caused a massive increase in weight, and this was probably due to alterations in the gut flora of the mice.

Now I am not saying that everybody is obese because they take too many antibiotics and have abnormal gut flora. Weight gain and metabolic syndrome are definitely multifactorial. I would, however, like to caution you all from taking masses of antibiotics for colds and coughs, which is bad medicine after all, and may make you fat on the inside and on the outside to boot!

DON'T EAT CARBOHYDRATES LATE AT NIGHT

This one is pretty obvious: don't eat too much before you go to sleep, especially if what you are eating is full of carbohydrates, which will cause a release of insulin into your bloodstream, allowing your body to store all those calories as fat while you slumber. If you need to snack, hit a lean protein instead; it will keep you satisfied and keep your blood insulin levels under control.

If you are heavy and trying to shed some of those pounds, you will undoubtedly know about the new weight-loss drugs and surgeries that curb your appetite or change your anatomy, all in an effort to make you trim. I, personally, don't prescribe any of these drugs to my patients because I focus on sleep, food, exercise and stress. And luckily for me, I have plenty of friendly colleagues who are happy to oversee the use of these medications. I do, however, want to tell you what the most current research says about these new antiobesity drugs and inform you of the potential problems you might encounter if you decide to try them.

In November 2013, scientists from the National Institutes of Health reviewed the results of 21 weight-loss drug studies in the prestigious *Journal of the American Medical Association*. They concluded that when the medications were taken in conjunction with diet and exercise, the average drop in body weight was between 3 and 9 percent. That is pretty good, and I am delighted to see that it wasn't just taking a pill that worked; you have to commit to a lifestyle change, as you all have done, to see the magic work. So there can be no doubt that these drugs work. However, nothing in life is risk-free, so here are some of the well-known side effects and concerns about our new friends.

Xenical and Alli work by keeping your gut from absorbing the fat you eat. They can therefore cause bloating and oily stools. Not a big deal in my opinion, and, frankly, if the inevitable bloating makes you think twice about that pepperoni pizza with extra cheese, then this could be a good option for you.

Qnexa appears to reduce appetite and food cravings, but it can cause cleft palates, or hare lips, in babies whose mothers take this medication. As this is the Man Diet, I am not concerned that you might become pregnant and have a deformed child, so this product may also be one to consider if you are struggling.

Finally, Belviq appears to work on the satiety area of the brain, reducing your appetite by telling you that you are full. The concern with this drug is that it is similar in chemical structure to fenfluramine, aka fen-phen, the diet pill that caused heart problems in the 1990s.

For those of you who prefer a more radical approach than a daily pill, there are different types of weight-loss surgeries that can either shrink your stomach using a band or even remove part of your stomach, all in an effort to make you feel full quicker and eat less.

Make no mistake, my friends, these surgeries definitely work and can significantly improve your diabetes very quickly after the procedure. The down side is that everybody knows someone who has put all the weight back on after undergoing one of these procedures. Also this is surgery, after all; doctors will be cutting you open, so there is always a risk of things going very wrong, even if it is a small one.

THREE MYTHS AND EIGHT FACTS ABOUT OBESITY THAT YOU NEED TO KNOW

The number one myth is a good one. Gentlemen, for 10 points, true or false?

Sex burns 300 calories.

And the answer is....................................FALSE (it is more like 150 calories per half an hour of romance!)

But don't take my word for it. Let's just look at a study published in the world's most prestigious medical journal, the *New England Journal of Medicine.* In January 2013, scientists at the University of Alabama published a paper after they had searched press reports and scientific writings on dieting, obesity and weight gain. The first thing they concluded was that there were lots of false and unproven claims. The number of calories we expend during sex was one of the myths that they exploded.

Another myth is that cutting just a few calories out of your diet every day has a significant impact on long-term weight loss. I think we all realize that a lifestyle makeover requires a significant change from your current dietary intake, and that's why my diet takes over 700 calories out of your diet every day.

How about the theory that if you lose a lot of weight fast you are more likely to put it back on than if you do it gradually? That one turns out to be a myth too—which is good for you because I'm aiming for most of you to drop 20–30 pounds (9–13.5 kg) in only twelve weeks!

And now for the eight facts:

- Genes are a large contributor to obesity, but they can be overcome by serious lifestyle changes.
- Calories in versus calories out matters.
- Exercise is good for you (seriously, dude, way to state the obvious).
- Exercise is a weight-maintenance tool.
- Your kids will lose weight if they see you living a healthy lifestyle.

- Structured meals (Jenny Craig, NutriSystem) and meal replacement plans (Medifast) do work (I just prefer you to eat fresh food, not packaged meals, and real food, not fake food bars).
- Weight-loss drugs work.
- Bariatric surgery works too!

Now to an issue that I see all too often and which can decimate all your hard-won successes in a single night of carnage: Binge eating.

BINGE EATING: FINALLY THERE IS HELP AT HAND!

Binge eating is the uncontrollable urge to eat as much as you can. It is not really related to hunger, but rather it is an emotional type of eating. Most people who binge eat may not even be aware that they are eating as much as they are during a binge period. This isn't about appetite or even feeling full. Binge eaters are eating to console themselves and using food for comfort rather than fuel. It is an emotion rather than hunger that is making them binge. Food is an ally and an enemy all at once, and the act of eating is stressful and filled with struggle and anxiety.

Everybody enjoys a meal with good friends around a sunny table in a joyful atmosphere. It must be terrible to be a binge eater who finds every mealtime a challenge filled with such intense emotions as love and hate.

Many of my patients are binge eaters. They usually confess to this after a while because they want to stop. The first step to recovery from every disease is to acknowledge that you have the disease.

No one can stick to any diet if he or she is depressed. Imagine trying to diet if you are a binge eater! You may be able to stick to a program for a short time, but eventually your underlying daily battle of emotions and food will get the better of you, and you'll fall off the wagon. Sorry to sound so bleak, but this is an issue that can't be swept under the carpet. It will sneak back out eventually. So what can we do about this problem?

We can learn a cutting-edge technique called mindfulness-based eating (MB-EAT) that helps change peoples' relationship with food. The technique is based on the work of one of the leading figures in the world of integrative medicine, John Kabat-Zinn, from the University of Massachusetts.

When you put on your socks every day, do you start with the right or left? Have you ever found yourself getting to work by car and not being able to recall anything about the drive you just completed? We live a lot of our lives on auto-pilot, doing many mundane activities like dressing, driving or even eating in a trancelike, automatic fashion, really not aware of what we are doing. If you were to perform one of these tasks with the full awareness of what you were doing, that would be called mindfulness.

Mindfulness really means concentrating and focusing all of your attention on the task or activity that you are performing. It is a form of meditation. When elite athletes are in the zone during a game, totally focused, not distracted by anything, they are in a state of mindfulness.

Now imagine eating with mindfulness, with total focus, concentrating on the texture, taste and smell of every bite. Eating slowly and savoring every instant! That is one of the core components of MB-EAT, and it is much harder than it sounds!

Clearly MB-EAT is the polar opposite of the mindless binge eating that some people fall into when they are upset. MB-EAT teaches people to cultivate awareness of what being hungry and being full really feels like. It helps you recognize why you are eating. Are you eating because you are hungry or are eating because you are actually upset and looking for love?

Other vital components of MB-EAT are the concepts of self-acceptance and wisdom. Participants in the program are encouraged to recognize that they have an internal wisdom, a guide that can give them helpful advice to cope with their difficulties. They learn self-acceptance and how to forgive themselves, learning to ignore the negative thoughts about themselves that pop into their heads when they are faced with food challenges.

It may sound rather New Age, but there is growing evidence that this technique actually works for people who are binge eaters. In one study, 18 morbidly obese women who had been diagnosed with binge-eating disorder participated in seven sessions of MB-EAT over a six-week period. At the end of the program, the number of weekly binges had dropped by nearly 75 percent (from four weekly binges per person to just over one). In addition, the patients all stated that they were eating significantly less food during their remaining binges compared to before the program.

Want to learn more?

There are many integrative medicine centers around the country that offer MB-EAT courses, including ours. Using Google to search for a course near to you is a good way to start. Alternatively, you could come and visit us in picturesque Connecticut—we would love to see you here!

I am finishing off this section by answering the most common question that I am asked by my patients on this diet:

"I lost twenty pounds (9-kg) and now I can't seem to lose any more. Have I reached a plateau?"

"Ah. The dreaded plateau," I reply.

Unfortunately, it is real and there are some very good reasons why it happens.

THE PLATEAU PHASE

In my opinion, the most critical reason people plateau is a case of simple math.

On August 27, 2011, researchers at the National Institute of Diabetes and Digestive and Kidney Diseases in Bethesda, Maryland, published an article in *The Lancet*. What they proposed was groundbreaking.

Most of us are aware of the simple weight-loss math that states that to lose one pound (454 g) of fat, you need to burn off an extra 3,500 calories. Since most diets set the number of calories you eat by about 500 less than what you need per day, it will take you approximately seven days, or one week, to lose that pesky pound (454 g). (500 calories per day × 7 days = 3,500 calories lost over a week). All good so far?

So, according to that simple math, if you are keeping to a diet that is at least 500 calories less than what your daily caloric needs are, then every week you'll lose one pound (454 g), and over one year (there are 52 weeks in a year) you will lose roughly 50 pounds (22.7 kg).

Now for the earth-shattering news flash.

According to *The Lancet* article, these standard weight-loss rules, endorsed by the National Institutes of Health and the American Diabetes Association are wrong!

To quote the researchers, "Common rules of thumb exaggerate how much weight people will lose from a given dietary calorie reduction, leading to unrealistic expectations and disappointment."

How can this be, you may be asking yourself. What is wrong with the pound-per-week rule?

Well, dear friends. What is wrong with the pound-per-week rule is that the math doesn't add up. Let me explain.

Everybody needs to eat a certain number of calories per day just to keep things running smoothly. The body has many, many functions and processes going on day and night, and they all need to be fueled by energy— energy that comes from food.

Depending on your weight, you will need between 1,700 and 2,000 calories per day just to keep things functioning. This is sometimes called your resting metabolic rate (RMR). The more you weigh, the more of you there is to feed, and the higher your daily requirements (RMR) will be.

Men are usually larger and heavier than women, so their daily RMR is likely to be higher to begin with.

Now for the math issue.

The problem with the pound-per-week rule of thumb is that it assumes that your RMR doesn't change as you lose weight. But according to the researchers, it does. Permit me to illustrate the point, and you'll see exactly what I mean.

Imagine a middle-aged man who is 30 pounds (13.6 kg) overweight. Unfortunately, not an uncommon phenomenon in today's America. Let's say he starts off with an RMR of 2,000 calories per day. He then goes on a 1,500 calorie per day diet, which is 500 calories less than what he needs every day. So he loses weight. Great!

After five months (20 weeks), he has lost 20 pounds (9 kg). *Mazel tov*! But something has changed. His RMR has gone down. There is less of him that needs to be fed now, so he doesn't need 2,000 calories per day, he only needs 1,700. The goalpost has moved as his body has slimmed down.

If he is still on the same 1,500 calorie per day diet, he won't be eating 500 calories less than what he needs; he will now be eating 200 calories less than what he needs (1,700 – 1,500 = 200). As you can obviously see, if you are eating 200 calories per day less than you need, then you will lose weight much, much more slowly.

In fact, the researchers from Bethesda calculated that because "human metabolism responds dynamically to changes in diet and body composition," losing 50 pounds (22.7 kg) would take three years rather than the usual one year that everybody believes it does.

That's the math, folks. And that's why, as you get closer to your goal weight, your weight loss can slow down and you can plateau.

What to do, what to do?

The answer is very simple. You need to increase your daily metabolic requirements so that you continue to eat at least 500 calories less than you need, even as your weight drops and your RMR goes down. The healthiest and safest way to increase your metabolic rate is through exercise, which I think we all know.

I have one more nugget to share about the plateau, and we will close out this section. (Sorry it is so long, but this is where you get the secrets to succeeding on my eating plan.) If you deviate more than infrequently from my eating plan, you will stop losing weight. As I said before, you are aiming to be good about 85–90 percent of the time.

I have used this diet with more than 10,000 people, and I can honestly say that it will not work properly if you don't do it properly.

Being on the program 50 percent of the time may reap some mild benefits, but if you want to really lose weight and significantly drop your sugar and cholesterol levels, you need to keep to this path faithfully.

Sometimes people stop losing weight and can't work out why. If this happens to you, my advice is to use an online food journal (like MyPlate at livestrong.com or MyFitnessPal, which we talked about at the beginning of this section) to help you identify those extra hidden calories that you didn't know you were eating. It is very enlightening to see what you are actually eating. You can use an online tool or smartphone application, to help you correct what you are doing in order to get back on track.

Just remember, a plateau is a slowing down, not a stop, so if you keep to the plan, you'll get there, I promise. I've seen thousands of people succeed using my approach. I have no doubt that you will too, with a little help from the practical pearls of wisdom in this section.

KEEPING IT GOING FOR THE LONG HAUL

Congratulations! You can finally close your trousers with ease and fit into the pair of pants you wore on your wedding day. And the other amazing achievement is that, when you go back to your doctors, they will be both delighted and amazed by the fact that your sugar level is now normal again and your cholesterol level has returned to the level it was when you were sixteen.

This is not a fantasy, I see this every single day in my clinical practice. In fact, a bad day for me is when the combined weight loss of all the patients I see on that day is less than 100 pounds (45 kg). In the three years that I've worked in private practice in Greenwich, Connecticut, I can count on one hand the number of patients I needed to start on a cholesterol-lowering or a sugar-lowering medication.

And by the way, there's nothing particularly unusual or out of the ordinary about the patients I see. They are just like you. They are overweight, tired and worried, even desperate. They want to feel better, look slimmer and avoid taking pills for the rest of their life. So they come to see me and just do what I instruct them to do. Do they fall off the wagon from time to time? For sure! But what sets them apart from the others is that they climb back up and continue riding toward their new future. Eventually they get there. And don't forget that you can enjoy the 60 recipes that Gav described in his section, so you'll see that this is entirely doable.

This next section is about how to keep the weight from ever coming back. It also gives you ways to keep your cholesterol and sugar levels in the normal range that they are in now.

Keeping weight off and the levels down isn't easy, and we will talk about the science behind why that is.

But first, let's look at three different options that you have for modifying your eating plan so that you don't return to that place of fat and fatigue, high sugar, cholesterol and frustration, where you used to be.

OPTION 1

Slowly and carefully reintroduce low glycemic index starches into your diet. But remember that this is a dangerous thing to do because before you know it, things could snowball out of control and you'll be back to the way you used to eat with your weight, cholesterol and sugar levels back up to where they used to be. The low glycemic index starches that I am talking about are foods like quinoa, yams, brown rice or whole wheat pasta, cooked al dente.

If you are going to eat them again, stick to no more than two servings of the low glycemic index starches per week. Just so you are clear about all of this, one sweet, medium-sized yam, or half a cup (95 g) of cooked rice, pasta or quinoa is a reasonable serving size.

Bread is a little bit trickier because people seem to go on feeding frenzies with bread, and it all goes wrong quickly. If you want to eat a slice of bread every two to three days, pick a whole-grain variety that is packed with seeds and that will invariably take your gut a long time to digest. I have found that European-style bakeries sometimes offer very dense whole-grain loaves. This hardy food harkens back to a time when bread was bread and people were still active enough to need it.

Remember, you are eating starch again and eating starch is a privilege, which comes with a responsibility: you must burn it off with physical activity. This is the maintenance phase, and as I have said before, exercise is a weight-maintenance tool, so you need to be using it to keep your weight stable and your numbers normal.

Is there any data to back up my recommendations? Why yes, there is. Sort of.

We shall now look at a trial that used intermittent carbohydrate restriction with 114 overweight or obese ladies over a three-month period and see how they fared on their journey to wellness.

This study comes from across the pond in merry England and was presented at the San Antonio Breast Cancer Symposium in December 2011.

The women were divided into three groups. The women in group number one ate only 600 calories a day on two days of the week. They achieved this difficult feat by cutting down their total carbohydrate intake to only 40 grams on those days (just to remind you, my diet has at least 100 grams of carbohydrate per day, which makes it a lot easier to handle). On the other five days of the week, they could eat whatever they liked, starches and all!

Group number two had a slightly different variation on the low-carb theme. The women in this group ate a healthy Mediterranean diet for five days of the week, switching to a low-carb diet for the other two days.

Sound familiar? This is a variation of the option for modifying my diet, which I have described to you: slowly reintroducing low glycemic index good starches back into your diet. I should point out, though, that there is a critical difference between what this group did and what I am proposing that you do. I am recommending that you eat a Mediterranean-style diet with high-quality starches only twice per week and stick to my reduced-starch plan for the other five days. This study group did the reverse of what I am suggesting: they ate starches for five days and none for two.

The third group just ate a 1,500 calorie per day, healthy Mediterranean diet without any weekly starving or carb deprivations!

What happened after three months?

Women in groups one and two, the low-carb-only and the low-carb and caloric restriction groups, had a significantly greater decline in markers for insulin resistance compared to the ladies who stuck to the 1,500 calorie per day Mediterranean feast.

The way I see it is that, although the women in this study certainly ate high-quality starches on more days of the week than I would recommend, forgoing starches on only two days of the week still led to a significant improvement on their blood glucose level.

Now you can understand why reintroducing low glycemic index starch back into your diet in a controlled and limited way works to keep things under control.

Incidentally, this study is a very beautiful segue into the second option for keeping your weight, sugar and cholesterol under control: intermittent fasting (alternating between periods of eating normally and periods of drinking just water, not juice).

As you can well imagine, the concept of intermittent fasting is similar to the diet of the ladies in the study who ate only 600 calories of a low-carb fare on two days of week. And their sugar levels turned out great too!

OPTION 2

This option allows you to eat more of what you want during the week, but once per week you adopt a regular 24-hour fasting habit to help compensate for dietary indiscretions.

This may not be as strange as it seems when you remember that regular fasting is very common in Mediterranean countries, and there are some health benefits to regularly drinking only liquids for a 24-hour period.

Studies have shown that intermittent fasting can reduce your blood glucose, weight and cholesterol and can provide many other health benefits, including possibly even making you live longer! You see, it turns out that one of the only ways to increase the life expectancy of mammals (which we all are) is by restricting their calories.

Don't believe me? Check this out.

In July 2009, Dr. Richard Weindruch and colleagues at the University of Wisconsin reported the results of a 20-year study on macaque monkeys in the prestigious journal *Science*. The trial began in 1989 when the researchers obtained 76 animals. These furry primates were divided into two groups: a control group who received a healthy diet that included all the essential nutrients that growing monkeys need, and an intervention group who had an identical diet but with 30 percent fewer calories.

Remember folks, that's two decades of being fed 30 percent less food than your friends! Sounds tough. Sounds like it would have started a monkey war to me! But rest assured, it didn't, and the results of the study are astonishing.

Only 60 percent of the original monkeys who ate a normal number of calories were still alive after 20 years compared to almost 90 percent of those who were on the continuous calorically restricted diet.

Here are the other stats, so you can see what fasting can do for you, even if you aren't furry:

Of the animals on the regular diet, 13 percent developed diabetes and 29 percent were classified as prediabetic after twenty years. Would you like to guess how many of the monkeys on the calorically restricted diet developed prediabetes or even frank diabetes? Not one. Even those who had sugar issues at the start of the study never developed prediabetes or diabetes, unlike their fully fed friends in the other group.

The incidence of any cancer in the calorically restricted group was half the rate seen in the animals on the regular diet.

Finally, the incidence of heart disease was reduced by half in the calorically restricted monkeys, compared to the controls.

The researchers concluded that the monkeys who ate 30 percent fewer calories for the entire 20-year period were biologically younger than their counterparts.

The bottom line, ladies and gentleman, is that eating 30 percent less food forever is a tall order for most of us but may actually extend your life. I hope that it now becomes clearer to you why a weekly fasting practice may help keep the pounds off and the blood test results positive.

OPTION 3

The third option that you have before you is to increase the amount of protein that you eat as long as the protein is still of the lean variety.

Personally, this is the approach that I tend to follow. I'm not a huge bread addict anyway, so I prefer extra helpings of white meat, tofu, fish or fat-free Greek yogurt with nuts and 85 percent dark chocolate! Doesn't sound too bad, right?

One advantage of this approach is the thermic effect of protein, which I talked about before and means that, because protein is an inefficient fuel source compared to carbohydrates, eating more of it will help burn off more calories compared to eating lots of starchy carbs.

There is another advantage to the increased protein option: it turns out that eating diets high in protein causes you to feel satiated faster. So, putting it another way, eating more protein can make you full quicker, therefore you may end up eating less food at each meal.

And here is one more good thing about eating lots of protein. It turns out that eating a high-protein diet will increase your lean muscle mass. Here is the study to illustrate my point.

The study was published in the *Journal of the American Medical Association* in January 2012. Researchers in Louisiana took 25 young men and women and housed them and overfed them by 1,000 calories per day for two months! (The things that people will do for free food and shelter!)

The really clever thing about the study was that the researchers varied the amount of protein they gave to different members of the group. Some people got a diet that was 25 percent protein (which is slightly higher than the 15 percent protein diets of most Americans), others got the standard 15 percent and yet others were fed a diet where only 5 percent of their total daily calories came from protein.

The obvious result of feeding people an extra 1,000 calories per day for two months was that everybody put on weight. Not a great surprise. Everybody knows that if you eat too much, you put on weight. But here are some other results that may amaze and surprise you:

Those who ate the 5 percent protein diet put on seven pounds (3.2-kg). When their body composition was analyzed, one and a half pounds (0.7-kg) of the weight gain was from increased muscle and five and a half pounds (2.5-kg) was from extra fat. Clearly, then, eating a low-protein diet that is excessively high in calories puts on extra pounds, mostly pounds of fat. So what happened to the folks on the high-protein diet?

As they too were overeating by 1,000 calories per day, they also gained weight—a whopping fourteen pounds (6.3-kg) over two months. But when the body composition of these people was analyzed, seven pounds (3.2-kg) of the extra fourteen pounds (6.3-kg) of "love" that they had amassed was muscle. In other words, half the extra weight they all gained was due to an increase in muscle, not fat!

There are two take-home messages from this study:

- Eating too much guarantees that your body will pack on the same amount of fat, regardless of how much protein you eat.
- Eating a diet high in protein leads to an increase in lean muscle mass (muscle).

In summary, increasing your protein intake during the weight maintenance phase of my diet is clearly a reasonable option since it will make you more satiated, will have a thermogenic effect on your body and appears to increase lean muscle mass.

But is there such a thing as too much protein in a diet? Yes, is the straightforward answer. Let's look at the Atkins data, and you'll see exactly what I mean.

In 2010, researchers in Boston analyzed data from two very large population studies that had involved more than 85,000 women and over 44,000 men and had lasted for over 20 years. The question they were asking was whether low-carbohydrate, high–animal protein diets (à la Atkins) were associated with an increased risk of dying!

And would you believe the researchers found that those who eat a high-animal–protein, low-carbohydrate diet had between a 23 percent and a 37 percent increased risk of dying compared to those who eat a "regular diet?"

Now for the good news.

The same analysis showed that those who eat a high-vegetable, low-carbohydrate diet, which is similar to the Man Diet, had a 20 percent reduction in the risk of dying compared to those who eat a "regular diet."

Now my diet is a long way from Atkins, but this frightening study is certainly food for thought.

And so, the answer to the question of whether there is such a thing as too much protein is, You bet! Especially if it involves large amounts of animal protein that is high in saturated fat.

KEEPING THE WEIGHT OFF

We are coming to the end of this final section, and before I sign off I want to briefly talk about two very important topics. The first one is the answer to the following question:

What are the scientifically proven ways to keep the weight off once you've have lost it?

You see, you don't need to reinvent the wheel. If scientists have already researched what works and what doesn't, that might be a pretty useful bit of information to know, don't you think?

However, before I tell you about the four keys to keeping weight off, I want to introduce the second and even more critical question:

Even though I have gotten rid of my love handles, why is my appetite exactly same as it was when I was fat?

The answer to this question will take us back to our old friends leptin and ghrelin, the hormones that govern our appetite. I'll tell you about the latest research on how they can still affect your eating habits long after you are sleek and slim.

The four keys, as I like to call them, come from interviews during a Penn State study of over 1,200 adults who had all successfully lost at least 30 pounds (13.5 kg) and then kept them off for one year afterward.

Ladies and gentleman, boys and girls, here are the four keys;

- Eat plenty of low-fat protein (and wouldn't you know, that's what I just told you to do!)
- Reward yourself from time to time. It is OK to cheat, it is even recommended, but, again, remember to make it worth it, and don't do it often.
- Follow a consistent exercise program. As I said earlier in this chapter, exercise is an excellent weight maintenance tool. So use it!

And, finally . . .

- You will always need to be vigilant, reminding yourself that your weight has been an issue in the past and needs to be controlled.

I realize that this is a rather depressing thought. If you were once fat, it appears that you can never just forget about it and stop watching what you eat. Unfortunately, the truth is that your weight is going to be something you will have to watch from now on. Making sure that if the scale starts going north again, you reevaluate what you have been eating and check whether those three *S*s—starch, sugar and saturated fat— have sneaked their way back onto your plate.

Now back to the age-old dieters' question: "I lost 30 pounds (13.5 kg) already but I am still as hungry as I ever was. What on earth is going on?" The answer to this excellent enquiry was published in the *New England Journal of Medicine* in October 2011.

Researchers in Australia enrolled 50 overweight or obese patients for a ten-week weight-loss program that cut their calories to 500 per day! They basically starved for almost three months.

Needless to say, they all lost about 30 pounds (13.5 kg).

But what was cool about this particular study is that the scientists also measured levels of leptin and ghrelin and other hormones that control appetite. There results were as follows:

After ten weeks of eating 500 calories per day, which led to a 30-pound (13.5-kg) weight loss, the levels of leptin (the hormone that is made in fat cells and makes you feel full) in the bloodstream significantly dropped. This isn't a great surprise. If you are on a starvation diet, then you won't be feeling full a lot.

At the same time, the levels of ghrelin (the hormone that makes your tummy rumble when you are hungry) in the blood significantly increased. This is no small wonder either, because I imagine that these peoples' stomachs were rumbling all the time.

Here is the kicker.

The investigators continued to follow these participants for a whole year after they had lost all that weight. They found that the average person gained back 12 pounds (5.4 kg), which isn't too bad when you consider that they lost almost triple that amount in the first place. However, even after one year, the levels of leptin and ghrelin in the blood had not returned to the levels they were before the study.

These poor people were still fighting with their appetite more than a year after they stopped dieting because of the changes in the levels of these hormones in their bodies! The bottom line is that the body takes a long time to get used to a new weight, and it sometimes keeps fighting to pack the pounds on again.

Weight loss is a long battle, and this unfortunate research shows that the fight isn't over just because you have reached your weight-loss goal. On the contrary, the fight is still very much on.

And just before I end the book, I want to ask you to step up to the plate. In this book, I have referred to two clinical studies that used the Man Diet approach to lower weight, cholesterol and blood glucose levels in men. I want to now briefly tell you about a new study I am doing to show how effective the Man Diet really is. This time, however, you are the trial participant. I want your data!

If you decide to try my lifestyle plan, please email CJFeuerstein@stamhealth.org your results (height, weight, blood pressure, cholesterol and blood glucose levels) at the beginning and after 10 to 12 weeks. You can get a copy of your labs from your MD—they belong to you!

What I am aiming to do is get the results from 3,000 to 5,000 men, and then publish all their data in a final huge study that will really prove to patients and doctors alike that the Man Diet is the way to go. As a thank you for your participation, Gav and I will send you 20 new recipes to whet your appetite more!

Rest assured, all your results will be kept totally confidential and no one will be able to access them except me and my team of trained researchers. In addition, any of your results that are published in a medical journal will be de-identified, which means that any features that could identify you will be removed.

So join the revolution to make the world thinner on the inside and the out!

I would like to end this book by saying to you what I have said to at least 10,000 people so far, as they embarked upon this new journey: You may find this difficult for about five days as your body gets used to living without so much starch, and even after that it may not all be smooth sailing, but I guarantee you'll see the results you seek.

The Man Diet is your personal guide to a newer, better you.

ACKNOWLEDGMENTS

There are many people I should thank for their help and guidance including the staff at the Boyd Center in Greenwich Connecticut, and the Center for Integrative Medicine at Stamford Hospital.

This dietary approach has entailed hours of phone calls with patients, something that would be impossible to do in a busy practice without the help of medical assistants, front desk-staff, nurses and a myriad of other people who have helped me along the way. This book is truly a testament to their hard work and faith in me.

On a personal note, I'm truly grateful to my family for their understanding and patience. I imagine they all wondered when this would finally be over and I realize that the time I spent with this project was time away from them. Gav and I would like to express "only love" for Marilyn Allen, our literary agent, and Page Street Publishing for believing in this diet revolution.

I offer thanks to my creator for guiding me in this journey and for being my companion and guardian.

Finally, there is no doubt that this was a team effort and I truly want to thank the thousands of patients that help me shape this diet, sticking to it despite the lack of comfort food! I salute every one of you and every pound you shed with me.

ABOUT THE AUTHORS

JOSEPH S. FEUERSTEIN, MD

Dr. Feuerstein was born in England and studied medicine at the University of London and Business Management at Cambridge University. He completed a rotating internship in general and trauma surgery at the Tel Aviv University Tel Hashomer teaching hospital before serving as combat physician in two elite units of the Israeli Navy (where he is still a reserve officer, with the rank of captain). He moved to the United States 13 years ago and completed an internship and residency in family medicine at the Columbia University/Stamford Hospital Family Medicine residency program, where he served as chief resident in his final year. He then spent two years studying with Dr. Andrew Weil as part of his fellowship in integrative medicine at the University of Arizona's School of Medicine.

He is currently the director of integrative medicine at Stamford Hospital, where for the last seven years he has run an insurance-based consultation service using nutrition, hypnosis, acupuncture, botanicals and stress management to help treat chronic medical problems such as obesity, diabetes, elevated cholesterol, hypertension, coronary heart disease, cancer, rheumatoid arthritis and depression. He has seen over 20,000 patients.

Dr. Feuerstein is an award-winning researcher in the field of clinical nutrition and herbal medicine, winning the 2015 Doctor of Excellence award from the Fairfield County Medical Society. As a result of full-time clinical activities and published research, Dr. Feuerstein has created the Man Diet program, based on 10,000 patients, and proven to work in two published clinical studies.

Dr. Feuerstein is an associate professor of clinical medicine at Columbia University and also works as a medical teaching attending at Greenwich Hospital.

He received certification in medical acupuncture from SUNY Downstate and is also certified in clinical hypnosis through two-year training under the American Society of Clinical Hypnosis. He holds a license as a homeopathic physician from the state of Connecticut. In September 2015, Dr. Feuerstein launched a monthly TV show on the Evine channel called *Optilife by Dr. Joe*, available in 83 million USA homes.

His other interests include daily aerobic exercise, Tai Chi, yoga and studying the Talmud.

Dr. Feuerstein lives in Weston, Connecticut with his wife, four children, three dogs, two cats and fish. You can learn more about Dr. Feuerstein by visiting his website drfeuerstein.com.

GAVIN PRITCHARD, RDN, CSSD, CD-N, CDE

Gavin Pritchard is an outpatient registered dietitian with Population Health and Prevention at Stamford Hospital. Gavin focuses on sports nutrition and risk reduction for chronic diseases such as obesity, heart disease and diabetes. He is a seasoned nutritionist and health supportive chef who has the unique ability to effectively guide individuals, families and groups toward their goals with personalized approaches to nutrition planning, menu creation and shopping, and improving health-supportive cooking skills.

Gavin earned his bachelor's degree in exercise science from the University of Colorado at Boulder. He completed his studies in nutrition at New York University and a yearlong internship at Yale-New Haven Hospital. Gavin has received advanced training in health-supportive cooking from the Culinary Institute of America in Hyde Park. He is also a board-certified sports specialist dietitian and a board-certified diabetes educator. He has earned advanced certification in adult, childhood and adolescent weight management.

REFERENCES

CHAPTER 1 REFERENCES

Aung, Koko, Carlos Lorenzo, Marco A. Hinojosa, and Steven M. Haffner. "Risk of Developing Diabetes and Cardiovascular Disease in Metabolically Unhealthy Normal-Weight and Metabolically Healthy Obese Individuals." *The Journal of Clinical Endocrinology & Metabolism* (2013): 462–468. doi:10.1210/jc.2013.2832.

Campbell, T. Colin, and Thomas M. Campbell. The China Study: The Most Comprehensive Study of Nutrition Ever Conducted and the Startling Implications for Diet, Weight Loss and Long-term Health. (Dallas, Texas: BenBella Books, 2005.)

Feuerstein, Joseph, Katherine Takayasu, Ashley Maltz, Wendy S. Bjerke, Hannah Hu, Izabel Nixon, and Caroline Mcquiston. "Teaching a Lifestyle Intervention for Reversing Impaired Fasting Glucose, Hyperlipidemia and Obesity/Overweight to a Cohort of Local Physicians." *Current Nutrition & Food Science* CNF 11, no. 1 (2015): 65–69.

Feuerstein, Joseph S., Leyna T. Bautista, and Wendy S. Bjerke. "A Dietary Approach for Treating Dyslipidemia and Hyperglycemia." *Current Nutrition & Food Science* 7, no. 4 (2011): 271–274.

Harcombe, Z., J. S. Baker, S. M. Cooper, B. Davies, N. Sculthorpe, J. J. Dinicolantonio, and F. Grace. "Evidence from Randomised Controlled Trials Did Not Support the Introduction of Dietary Fat Guidelines in 1977 and 1983: A Systematic Review and Meta-analysis." *Open Heart* 2, no. 1 (2015). doi:10.1136/openhrt-2014-000196.

Hu, Frank et al. "Dietary Fat Intake and the Risk of Coronary Heart Disease in Women." *New England Journal of Medicine* 337, no. 21 (1997): 1491–1499. doi:10.1056/NEJM199711203372102.

Jebb, Susan A., Amy L. Ahern, Ashley D. Olson, Louise M. Aston, Christina Holzapfel, Julia Stoll, Ulrike Amann-Gassner, Annie E. Simpson, Nicholas R. Fuller, Suzanne Pearson, Namson S. Lau, Adrian P. Mander, Hans Hauner, and Ian D. Caterson. "Primary Care Referral to a Commercial Provider for Weight Loss Treatment versus Standard Care: A Randomised Controlled Trial." *The Lancet* 378, no. 9801 (2011): 1485–1492. doi:10.1016/S0140-6736(11)61344-5.

Jenkins, D. J. A., J. M. W. Wong, C. W. C. Kendall, A. Esfahani, V. W. Y. Ng, T. C. K. Leong, D. A. Faulkner, E. Vidgen, K. A. Greaves, G. Paul, and W. Singer. "The Effect Of A Plant-Based Low-Carbohydrate ("Eco-Atkins") Diet on Body Weight and Blood Lipid Concentrations in Hyperlipidemic Subjects." *Archives of Internal Medicine* 169, no. 11 (2009): 1046–1054.

Lagiou, P., S. Sandin, M. Lof, D. Trichopoulos, H.O. Adami, and E. Weiderpass. "Low Carbohydrate—High Protein Diet and Incidence of Cardiovascular Diseases in Swedish Women: Prospective Cohort Study." *British Medical Journal* 344 (2012). doi:10.1136/bmi.e4026.

Mozaffarian, Dariush, Tao Hao, Eric B. Rimm, Walter C. Willett, and Frank B. Hu. "Changes in Diet and Lifestyle and Long-Term Weight Gain in Women and Men." *New England Journal of Medicine* (2011): 2392–2404.

Muraki, I., F. Imamura, J. E. Manson, F. B. Hu, W. C. Willett, R. M. Van Dam, and Q. Sun. "Fruit Consumption and Risk of Type 2 Diabetes: Results from Three Prospective Longitudinal Cohort Studies." BMJ (2013): F5001. doi:http//dx.doi.org/10.1136.bmj.f5001.

Renaud, S. "Wine, Alcohol, Platelets, and the French Paradox for Coronary Heart Disease." *The Lancet* 309, no. 8808 (1992): 1523–1526.

Ornish, D. "Can Lifestyle Changes Reverse Coronary Heart Disease? The Lifestyle Heart Trial." *The Lancet* 336, no. 8708 (1990): 129–133.

Sacks, Frank et al. "Comparison of Weight-Loss Diets with Different Compositions of Fat, Protein, and Carbohydrates." *The New England Journal of Medicine* 360 (2009): 859-873. doi:10.1056/NEJMoa0804748.

Schwarzfuchs, Dan, Rachel Golan, and Iris Shai. "Four-Year Follow-Up after Two-Year Dietary Interventions." *The New England Journal of Medicine* 367 (2012): 1373–1374.

Shai, Iris. "Weight Loss with a Low-Carbohydrate, Mediterranean, or Low-Fat Diet." *The New England Journal of Medicine* 359 (2008): 229–241.

Siri-Tarino, P. W, Q. Sun, F. B Hu, and R. M Krauss. "Meta-Analysis of Prospective Cohort Studies Evaluating the Association of Saturated Fat with Cardiovascular Disease." *American Journal of Clinical Nutrition* (2010): 535–546. doi:10.3945/ajcn.2009.27725.

Sugiyama, Takehiro, Yusuke Tsugawa, Chi-Hong Tseng, Yasuki Kobayashi, and Martin F. Shapiro. "Different Time Trends of Caloric and Fat Intake between Statin Users and Nonusers among US Adults." *JAMA Internal Medicine* JAMA Intern Med (2014): 1038. doi:10.1001/jamainternmed.2014.1927.

Sun, Q., D. Spiegelman, R. M. Van Dam, M. D. Holmes, V. S. Malik, W. C. Willett, and F. B. Hu. "White Rice, Brown Rice, and Risk of Type 2 Diabetes in US Men and Women." *Archives of Internal Medicine* 170, no. 11 (2010): 961–969.

Thompson, R.C. et al. "Atherosclerosis across 4000 Years of Human History: The Horus Study of Four Ancient Populations." *The Lancet* 381, no. 9873 (2013): 1211–1222. doi:SO140-6736(13)60598-X.

"Vital Signs: Prevalence, Treatment, and Control of High Levels of Low-Density Lipoprotein Cholesterol—United States, 1999–2002 and 2005–2008." *Morbidity and Mortality Weekly Report* 60, no. 4 (2011): 109–114.

Wang, Jingzhou, Bibiana García-Bailo, Daiva E. Nielsen, Ahmed El-Sohemy, and Nick Ashton. "ABO Genotype, 'Blood-Type' Diet and Cardiometabolic Risk Factors." *PLOS ONE* (2014): E84749. doi:10.1371/journal.pone.0084749.

Yang, Quanhe, Zefeng Zhang, Edward W. Gregg, W. Dana Flanders, Robert Merritt, and Frank B. Hu. "Added Sugar Intake and Cardiovascular Diseases Mortality among US Adults." *JAMA Internal Medicine JAMA Intern Med* (2014): 516. doi:10.1001/jamainternmed.2013.12991.

CHAPTER 2 REFERENCES

Ackerman, R.T. et al. "Identifying Adults at High Risk for Diabetes and Cardiovascular Disease Using Hemoglobin A1c National Health and Nutrition Examination Survey 2005–2006." *American Journal of Preventive Medicine* (2011): 11–17. doi:10.1016/j.amepre.2010.09.022.

Al-Shuwaykh, Harith. "Impaired Fasting Glucose (IFG) as a Risk Factor for Coronary Artery Disease (Cad) Compared to Diabetes Mellitus (DM) and Normal Blood Sugar in Association with Other Cad Risks." *American Association of Clinical Endocrinologists* Abstract 257 (2013).

Baudrand, R. et al. "High Sodium Intake Is Associated with Increased Glucocorticoid Production, Insulin Resistance and Metabolic Syndrome." *Clinical Endocrinology* 80, no. 5 (2014): 677-684. doi:10.1111/cen.12225.

Bleys, J. "Serum Selenium Levels and All-Cause, Cancer and Cardiovascular Mortality among US Adults." *Archives of Internal Medicine* 168, no. 4 (2008): 404–410.

Cheng, P., B. Neugaard, P. Foulis, and P. R. Conlin. "Hemoglobin A1c as a Predictor of Incident Diabetes." *Diabetes Care* 43, no. 3 (2011): 610–615. doi:10.2337/dc10-0625.

Contois, J. H. et al. "Apolipoprotein B and Cardiovascular Disease Risk: Position Statement from the AACC Lipoproteins and Vascular Diseases Division Working Group on Best Practices." *Clinical Chemistry* 55, no. 3 (2009): 407–419. doi:10.1373/clinchem.2008.118356.

De Smet, M. et al. "Short-Term Changes in Serum Sex Steroid Levels and Cardiac Function in Healthy Young Men." *European Congress of Endocrinology* (2013). doi:10.1530/endoabs.32.P182.

Dhindsa, S. "Testosterone Replacement Decreases Insulin Resistance in Hypogonadal Men with Type 2 Diabetes." *ENDO* Abstract (2013).

DRI Dietary Reference Intakes for Vitamin A, Vitamin K, Arsenic, Boron, Chromium, Copper, Iodine, Iron, Manganese, Molybdenum, Nickel, Silicon, Vanadium, and Zinc : A Report of the Panel on Micronutrients ... and the Standing Committee on the Scientific E. Washington, D.C.: *National Academy Press*, 2001. 258–259.

Epel, E. et al. "Stress and Body Shape: Stress-Induced Cortisol Secretion Is Consistently Greater among Women with Central Fat." *Psychosomatic Medicine* 5 (2000): 623–632.

Finkle W. et al. "Increased Risk of Nonfatal Myocardial Infarction Following Testosterone Therapy Prescription in Men." *PLOS One* Abstract (2014). doi: 10.137/journal/pone.0085805

Gartner, R. et al. "Selenium Supplementation in Patients with Auto-immune Thyroiditis Decreases Thyroid Peroxidase Antibody Concentrations." *The Journal of Clinical Endocrinology and Metabolism* 87, no. 4 (2002): 1687–1691.

Graudal, N. et al. "Compared with Usual Sodium Intake, Low- and Excessive-sodium Diets Are Associated with Increased Mortality: A Meta-analysis." *American Journal of Hypertension* 27, no. 9 (2014): 1129–1137. doi:10.1093/ajh/hpu028.

Hickman, Tamy B., Ronette R. Briefel, Margaret D. Carroll, Basil M. Rifkind, James I. Cleeman, Kurt R. Maurer, and Clifford L. Johnson. "Distributions and Trends of Serum Lipid Levels among United States Children and Adolescents Ages 4-19 Years: Data from the Third National Health and Nutrition Examination Survey." *Preventive Medicine* 27, no. 6 (1998): 879–890.

Hollowell J. et al. "Serum TSH, T4 and Thyroid antibodies in the United States Population (1988 to 1994): National Health and Nutrition Examination Survey (NHANES III)." *The Journal of Clinical Endocrinology and Metabolism* 87 no. 2 (2002): 489–499.

Laaksonen, D.E. et al. "Testosterone and Sex Hormone-binding Globulin Predict the Metabolic Syndrome and Diabetes in Middle-aged Men." *Diabetes Care* 27, no. 5 (2004): 1036–1041.

Lazzarino, A. et al. "The Association between Cortisol Response to Mental Stress and High Sensitivity Cardiac Troponin T Plasma Concentrations in Healthy Adults." *Journal of the American College of Cardiology* 62, no. 18 (2013): 1694–1701.

Otvos, J. D. "Clinical Implications of Discordance between Low-Density Lipoprotein Cholesterol and Particle Number." *Journal of Clinical Lipidology* (2011) 105–113. doi:10.1016/j.jacl.2011.02.001.

Rydén, L. et al. "ESC Guidelines on Diabetes, Prediabetes, and Cardiovascular Disease Developed in Collaboration with the EASD." *European Heart Journal* 34, no. 39 (2013): 3035–3087. doi:10.1093/eurheartj/eht108.

Razvi, S. et al. "Levothyroxine Treatment of Subclinical Hypothyroidism, Fatal and Nonfatal Cardiovascular Events, and Mortality." *Archives of Internal Medicine* 172, no. 10 (2012): 811–817. doi:10.1001/archinternmed.2012.1159.

Stone, N. et al. "2013 ACC/AHA Guideline on the Treatment of Blood Cholesterol to Reduce Atherosclerotic Cardiovascular Risk in Adults." 2013 ACC/AHA Guideline on the Treatment of Blood Cholesterol to Reduce Atherosclerotic Cardiovascular Risk in Adults 36, no. 25_PA (2014). doi:10.1016/j.jacc.2013.11.002.

"Stress, Hormones, and Weight Gain," Stöppler, M.C., accessed July 5, 2015, www.medicinenet.com/script/main/art.asp?articlekey=53304.

Thomson, C.D. et al. "Brazil Nuts: An Effective Way to Improve Selenium Status." *American Journal of Clinical Nutrition* 87, no. 2 (2008): 379–384.

Varbo, A. et al. "Nonfasting Triglycerides, Cholesterol, and Ischemic Stroke in the General Population." *Annals of Neurology* 69, no. 4 (2011): 628–634. doi:10.1002/ana.22384.

Veeranna, V. et al. "Homocysteine and Reclassification of Cardiovascular Disease Risk." *Journal of the American College of Cardiology* 58, no. 10 (2011): 1025–1033. doi:10.1016/j.jacc.2011.05.028.

Wilson, B. E., and A. Gondy. "Effects of Chromium Supplementation on Fasting Insulin Levels and Lipid Parameters in Healthy, Non-obese Young Subjects." *Diabetes Research and Clinical Practice*, 1995, 179–184.

Wu, T. et al. "Associations of Serum C-Reactive Protein with Fasting Insulin, Glucose, and Glycosylated Hemoglobin: The Third National Health and Nutrition Examination Survey, 1988–1994." *American Journal of Epidemiology* 155, no. 1 (2002): 65–71.

CHAPTER 3 REFERENCES

Belin, R. J., P. Greenland, L. Martin, A. Oberman, L. Tinker, J. Robinson, J. Larson, L. Van Horn, and D. Lloyd-Jones. "Fish Intake and the Risk of Incident Heart Failure: The Women's Health Initiative." *Circulation:* Heart Failure 4, no. 4 (2011): 404–413. doi:10.1161/CIRCHEARTFAILURE.110.960450.

Bernstein, A. M., Q. Sun, F. B. Hu, M. J. Stampfer, J. E. Manson, and W. C. Willett. "Major Dietary Protein Sources and Risk of Coronary Heart Disease in Women." *Circulation* 122, no. 9 (2010): 876–883.

Crowe, F. L. et al. "Fruit and Vegetable Intake and Mortality from Ischaemic Heart Disease: Results from the European Prospective Investigation into Cancer and Nutrition (EPIC)-Heart Study." *European Heart Journal* 32, no. 10 (2011): 1235–1243. doi:10.1093/eurheartj/ehq465.

Halton, T. L., and F. B. Hu. "The Effects of High Protein Diets on Thermogenesis, Satiety and Weight Loss: A Critical Review." *Journal of the American College of Nutrition* 23, no. 5 (2004): 373–385.

He, J., M. R. Wofford, K. Reynolds, J. Chen, C.-S. Chen, L. Myers, D. L. Minor, P. J. Elmer, D. W. Jones, and P. K. Whelton. "Effect of Dietary Protein Supplementation on Blood Pressure: A Randomized, Controlled Trial." *Circulation* 124, no. 5 (2011): 589–595. doi:10.1161/CIRCULATIONAHA.110.009159.

Mostofsky, E. et al. "Chocolate Intake and Incidence of Heart Failure: A Population-based Prospective Study of Middle-Aged and Elderly Women." *Circulation*: Heart Failure 3, no. 5 (2010): 612–616. doi: 10.1161/CIRCHEARTFAILURE.110.944025.

Park, Y., A. F. Subar, A. Hollenbeck, and A. Schatzkin. "Dietary Fiber Intake and Mortality in the NIH-AARP Diet and Health Study." *Archives of Internal Medicine* 171, no. 12 (2011): 1061–1068.

Salas-Salvado, J., J. Fernandez-Ballart, E. Ros, M.-A. Martinez-Gonzalez, M. Fito, R. Estruch, D. Corella, M. Fiol, E. Gomez-Gracia, F. Aros, G. Flores, J. Lapetra, R. Lamuela-Raventos, V. Ruiz-Gutierrez, M. Bullo, J. Basora, and M.-I. Covas. "Effect of a Mediterranean Diet Supplemented With Nuts on Metabolic Syndrome Status: One-Year Results of the PREDIMED Randomized Trial." *Archives of Internal Medicine* 168, no. 22 (2008): 2449–2458. doi:10.1001/archinte.168.22.2449.

Samieri, C., C. Feart, C. Proust-Lima, E. Peuchant, C. Tzourio, C. Stapf, C. Berr, and P. Barberger-Gateau. "Olive Oil Consumption, Plasma Oleic Acid, and Stroke Incidence: The Three-City Study." *Neurology* 77, no. 5 (2011): 418–425. doi:10.1212/WNL.0b013e318220abeb.

Smith-Spangler, C. et al. "Are Organic Foods Safer or Healthier than Conventional Alternatives?: A Systematic Review." *Annals of Internal Medicine* 157, no. 5 (2012): 348–366.

Trichopoulou, A., C. Bamia, and D. Trichopoulos. "Anatomy of Health Effects of Mediterranean Diet: Greek EPIC Prospective Cohort Study." *British Medical Journal,* 2009. doi: http://dx.doi.org/10.1136/bmj.b2337.

White House Task Force on Childhood Obesity Report to the President. "Solving the Problems of Childhood Obesity within a Generation." May 1, 2010.

CHAPTER 5 REFERENCES

Bateman, Lori A., Cris A. Slentz, Leslie H. Willis, A. Tamlyn Shields, Lucy W. Piner, Connie W. Bales, Joseph A. Houmard, and William E. Kraus. "Comparison of Aerobic versus Resistance Exercise Training Effects on Metabolic Syndrome (from the Studies oF A Targeted Risk Reduction Intervention through Defined Exercise - STRRIDE-AT/RT)." *The American Journal of Cardiology* 108, no. 6 (2011): 838–844.

Block, J. et al. "Consumers' Estimation of Calorie Content at Fast Food Restaurants: Cross Sectional Observational Study." *British Medical Journal,* 2013. doi: http://dx.doi.org/10.1136/bmj.f2907.

Bray, George A., Steven R. Smith, Lilian De Jonge, Hui Xie, Jennifer Rood, Corby K. Martin, Marlene Most, Courtney Brock, Susan Mancuso, and Leanne M. Redman. "Effect of Dietary Protein Content on Weight Gain, Energy Expenditure, and Body Composition during Overeating." *JAMA* 307, no. 1 (2012): 47–55.

Casazza, K. et al. "Myths, Presumptions, and Facts about Obesity." *New England Journal of Medicine* 368, no. 5 (2013): 446–454. doi:10.1056/NEJMsa1208051.

Colman, R. J., R. M. Anderson, S. C. Johnson, E. K. Kastman, K. J. Kosmatka, T. M. Beasley, D. B. Allison, C. Cruzen, H. A. Simmons, J. W. Kemnitz, and R. Weindruch. "Caloric Restriction Delays Disease Onset and Mortality in Rhesus Monkeys." *Science* 325, no. 5937 (2009): 201–204.

Ding, E. et al. "Randomized Trial of Social Network Lifestyle Intervention for Obesity: MICROCLINIC Intervention Results and 16-month Follow up." *American Heart Association,* 2013.

Elder, C. R., cup M Gullion, K. L. Funk, L. L. Debar, N. M. Lindberg, and V. J. Stevens. "Impact of Sleep, Screen Time, Depression and Stress on Weight Change in the Intensive Weight Loss Phase of the LIFE Study." *International Journal of Obesity* 36, no. 1 (2011): 86–92. doi:10.1038/ijo.2011.60.

Frisbee, Stephanie J., Anoop Shankar, Sarah S. Knox, Kyle Steenland, David A. Savitz, Tony Fletcher, and Alan M. Ducatman. "Perfluorooctanoic Acid, Perfluorooctanesulfonate, and Serum Lipids in Children and Adolescents." *Archives of Pediatrics & Adolescent Medicine* 164, no. 9 (2010): 860–869.

Fung, Teresa T. "Low-Carbohydrate Diets and All-Cause and Cause-Specific Mortality." *Annals of Internal Medicine* 153, no. 5 (2010): 289–298.

Gerche, A. La, A. T. Burns, D. J. Mooney, W. J. Inder, A. J. Taylor, J. Bogaert, A. I. Macisaac, H. Heidbuchel, and D. L. Prior. "Exercise-Induced Right Ventricular Dysfunction and Structural Remodelling in Endurance Athletes." *European Heart Journal* 33, no. 8 (2011): 998–1006. doi:10.1093/eurheartj/ehr397.

Hall, Kevin D, Gary Sacks, Dhruva Chandramohan, Carson cup Chow, Y Claire Wang, Steven L Gortmaker, and Boyd A Swinburn. "Quantification of the Effect of Energy Imbalance on Bodyweight." *The Lancet* 378, no. 9793 (2011): 826–837.

Harvie, M., C. Wright, M. Pegington, E. Mitchell, Dg Evans, S. Jebb, R. Clarke, R. Goodacre, W. Dunn, M. Mattson, and A. Howell. "P3-09-02: Intermittent Dietary Carbohydrate Restriction Enables Weight Loss and Reduces Breast Cancer Risk Biomarkers." Abstract presented at the San Antonio Breast Cancer Symposium, San Antonio, Texas, December 6–10, 2011.

Hoevenaar-Blom, M. P., A. M. Spijkerman, D. Kromhout, and W. M. Verschuren. "Sufficient Sleep Duration Contributes to Lower Cardiovascular Disease Risk in Addition to Four Traditional Lifestyle Factors: The MORGEN Study." *European Journal of Preventive Cardiology,* 2013. doi:10.1177/2047487313493057.

Howard, S., J. Adams, and M. White. "Nutritional Content of Supermarket Ready Meals and Recipes by Television Chefs in the United Kingdom: Cross Sectional Study." *British Medical Journal,* 2012. doi: http://dx.doi.org/10.1136/bmj.e7607.

Kennedy, Pagan. "The Fat Drug." *New York Times,* March 8, 2014.

Kokkinos, Alexander, Carel W. Le Roux, Kleopatra Alexiadou, Nicholas Tentolouris, Royce P. Vincent, Despoina Kyriaki, Despoina Perrea, Mohammad A. Ghatei, Stephen R. Bloom, and Nicholas Katsilambros. "Eating Slowly Increases the Postprandial Response of the Anorexigenic Gut Hormones, Peptide YY and Glucagon-Like Peptide-1." *The Journal of Clinical Endocrinology & Metabolism* 95, no. 1 (2009): 333–337. doi:10.1210/jc.2009-1018.

Kristeller, Jean L., and Ruth Q. Wolever. "Mindfulness-Based Eating Awareness Training for Treating Binge Eating Disorder: The Conceptual Foundation." *Eating Disorders* 19, no. 1 (2010): 49–61.

Laursen, A. H., O. P. Kristiansen, J. L. Marott, P. Schnohr, and E. Prescott. "Intensity versus Duration of Physical Activity: Implications for the Metabolic Syndrome. A Prospective Cohort Study." *British Medical Journal Open*, 2012. doi:10.1136/bmjopen-2012-001711.

Lee, I. M., L. Djousse, H. D. Sesso, L. Wang, and J. E. Buring. "Physical Activity and Weight Gain Prevention." *JAMA: The Journal of the American Medical Association* 303, no. 12 (2010): 1173–1179.

Lee, J. M. et al. "Bisphenol A and Chronic Disease Risk Factors in US Children." *Pediatrics*, 2013. doi:10.1542/peds.2013-0106.

Ma, Jun, Veronica Yank, Lan Xiao, Philip W. Lavori, Sandra R. Wilson, Lisa G. Rosas, and Randall S. Stafford. "Translating the Diabetes Prevention Program Lifestyle Intervention for Weight Loss into Primary Care." *JAMA Internal Medicine* 173, no. 2 (2013): 113–121. doi:10.1001/2013. jamainternmed.987.

Sciamanna, Christopher N., Michaela Kiernan, Barbara J. Rolls, Jarol Boan, Heather Stuckey, Donna Kephart, Carla K. Miller, Gordon Jensen, Terry J. Hartmann, Eric Loken, Kevin O. Hwang, Ronald J. Williams, Melissa A. Clark, Jane R. Schubart, Arthur M. Nezu, Erik Lehman, and Cheryl Dellasega. "Practices Associated with Weight Loss versus Weight-Loss Maintenance." *American Journal of Preventive Medicine* 41, no. 2 (2011): 159–166. doi:10.1016/j.amepre.2011.04.009.

Spring, B. et al. "Integrating Technology into Standard Weight Loss Treatment: A Randomized Control Trial." *JAMA Internal Medicine* 173, no. 2 (2013): 105–111. doi:10.1001/jamainternmed.2013.1221.

Srikanthan, P., and A. S. Karlamangla. "Relative Muscle Mass Is Inversely Associated with Insulin Resistance and Prediabetes. Findings from the Third National Health and Nutrition Examination Survey." *Journal of Clinical Endocrinology & Metabolism* 96, no. 9 (2011): 2898–2903. doi:10.1210/jc.2011-0435.

Sumithran, Priya, Luke A. Prendergast, Elizabeth Delbridge, Katrina Purcell, Arthur Shulkes, Adamandia Kriketos, and Joseph Proietto. "Long-Term Persistence of Hormonal Adaptations to Weight Loss." *New England Journal of Medicine* 365 (2011): 1597–1604.

Tal, Aner, and Brian Wansink. "Fattening Fasting: Hungry Grocery Shoppers Buy More Calories, Not More Food." *JAMA Internal Medicine* 173, no. 12 (2013): 1146–1148. doi:10.1001/jamainternmed.2013.650.

Tjønna, Arnt Erik, Ingeborg Megaard Leinan, Anette Thoresen Bartnes, Bjørn M. Jenssen, Martin J. Gibala, Richard A. Winett, Ulrik Wisløff, and Conrad P. Earnest. "Low- and High-Volume of Intensive Endurance Training Significantly Improves Maximal Oxygen Uptake after 10-Weeks of Training in Healthy Men." *PLoS ONE*, 2013. doi:10.1371/journal.pone.0065382.

Trasande, L., A. J. Spanier, S. Sathyanarayana, T. M. Attina, and J. Blustein. "Urinary Phthalates and Increased Insulin Resistance in Adolescents." *Pediatrics*, 2013. doi:10.1542/peds.2012-4022.

Urban, L. E., M. A. McCrory, G. E. Dallal, S. K. Das, E. Saltzman, J. L. Weber, and S. B. Roberts. "Accuracy of Stated Energy Contents of Restaurant Foods." *JAMA: The Journal of the American Medical Association* 306, no. 4 (2011): 287–293.

Wieland, L. Susan, Louise Falzon, Chris N Sciamanna, Kimberlee J Trudeau, Suzanne Brodney, Joseph E Schwartz, and Karina W Davidson. "Interactive Computer-Based Interventions for Weight Loss or Weight Maintenance in Overweight or Obese People." *Cochrane Database of Systematic Reviews*, 2012. doi:10.1002/14651858.CD007675.pub2.

Yanovski, Susan Z., and Jack A. Yanovski. "Long-Term Drug Treatment for Obesity: A Systematic and Clinical Review." *JAMA* 311, no. 1 (2013): 74–86. doi:10.1001/jama2013.281361.

INDEX

A

adrenal glands and cortisol, 46–50
aerobic exercise, study of, 182
All-Bran Buds, 54, 55, 76
Allspice-Rubbed Pork Tenderloin with Braised Red Cabbage and Grain Mustard, 86, *87*
Almonds, Toasted, and Roasted Pear with Cinnamon Ricotta, 168, *169*
American Association of Clinical Endocrinologists, 37
American College of Cardiology, 30, 31, 35, 38
American College of Sports Medicine, 181, 183
American Diabetes Association, 30, 31, 35, 189
American Heart Association, 15, 30, 175
American Journal of Cardiology, 182
American Journal of Clinical Nutrition, 18
American Journal of Hypertension, 50
Ancho Pork and Pinto Bean Stew, *88*, 89
antibiotics in animal feed, 186
apolipoproteins, 33
appetite
    controlled by hormones, 179–80, 185
    diet drugs, 187
    neuropeptides and, 185
    slow eating versus quick, 179–80
(Are You Kiddin' Me!) Crustless Quiche, 66, *67*
asparagus
    with Grilled Sweet Chili Pork Tenderloin, *100*, 101
    with Salmon "Steak" and Eggs and Lemon-Dill Yogurt Sauce, 80, *81*
Atkins diet, 20, 23, 24–25, 57, 194
avocado oils, 50, 58
avocados
    Avocado-Wasabi Dressing, for Baja Cobb Salad, 123
    Brocc-amole with Jicama, *152*, 153
    Buffalo Chicken Wedge with Buffalo Ranch Dressing, 126
    Fresh Start Salad, 75
    Grilled Chicken Enchilada with Summer Squash and Chili Roja, 98, *99*
    Santa Fe Chopped Salad with Smoky Ranch Dressing, *136*, 137
    South of the Border 7-Layer Parfait, *170*, 171

B

Baja Cobb Salad with Avocado-Wasabi Dressing, 123
Basic Baked Eggs, *70*, 71
BBQ Chicken Coleslaw, 125
beans, 58–59
    Ancho Pork and Pinto Bean Stew, *88*, 89
    (Are You Kiddin' Me!) Crustless Quiche, 66, *67*
    BBQ Chicken Coleslaw, *124*, 125
    black beans, 66, 69, 137, 171
    Devilish Eggs, 162, *163*
    green beans, 120, 132, 147
    Huevos Rancheros, 69

Ornish diet and, 18
pinto beans, 89
red kidney beans, 125
Santa Fe Chopped Salad with Smoky Ranch Dressing, *136*, 137
South of the Border 7-Layer Parfait, *170*, 171
beef
    extra-lean, 56
    Oven-Roasted Meatballs with Vegetable Caponata, *104*, 105
    Pan-Seared Beef Tenderloin with Shiitakes, Lemon and Parsley, 106, *107*
    Philly Cheesesteak Salad with Horsey Sauce, 135
    Rainbow Beef Stir-Fry, *108*, 109
    saturated fat and, 24
    Smoke-Signal Buffalo Chili, 116
berries
    Fresh Start Salad, *74*, 75
    Man Up Blueberry-Almond Muffins, *164*, 165
    Man Up Blueberry-Almond Muffins, *164*, 165
    raspberries in salad, *142*, 143
    Raspberry-Almond Mousse, 167
    Red, White and Blueberry Yogi Bowl, *78*, 79
    Summer Berry Fro-Yo Pops, 172, *173*
    as snack, 61
    as sweetener, 55, 59
binge eating, 188–90
Bison Hanger Steak with Chimichurri and Grilled Carrots, 90, *91*
bisphenol A (BPA) and obesity risk, 185
blood glucose levels, 10, 13, 14, 16–17, 20, 35–37, 50–51
blood pressure study, 58–59
blood tests
    apolipoprotein B levels, 29–35
    cardiac CRP, 37–38
    cholesterol, 29–38
    glycated hemoglobin (HbA1c) test, 19, 35–37
    LDL particle number, 29–35
    NMR LipoProfile, 30
blood-type diets, 25–26
body mass index (BMI) measurement of fat, 22, 39–40
body muscle mass and diabetes, 182
Braised Low-Country Pork Chops, 83
Braised Red Cabbage and Grain Mustard, with Allspice-Rubbed Pork Tenderloin, 86, *87*
bran, 54, 55, 76
breakfast, of Man Diet, 53–56
British Medical Journal, 24, 178
broccoli
    (Are You Kiddin' Me!) Crustless Quiche, 66
    Brocc-amole with Jicama, *152*, 153
    and levels of chromium, 51
    1-2-3 Scramble, 68
    Rainbow Beef Stir-Fry, 109

Roasted Veg Buddha Bowl with Tahini Dressing, 138
Brocc-amole with Jicama, *152*, 153
Buffalo Chicken Wedge with Buffalo Ranch Dressing, 126
Buffalo Legs, 154, *155*

C

cabbage
    Allspice-Rubbed Pork Tenderloin with Braised Red Cabbage and Grain Mustard, 86
    BBQ Chicken Coleslaw, 125
    Braised Red Cabbage and Grain Mustard, with Allspice-Rubbed Pork Tenderloin, 86, *87*
    Cheese and Snackers, 166
    Five-Spice Seared Salmon with Mu Shu Vegetables, 85
    Thai(riffic) Salmon Salad with Peanut-Lime Vinaigrette, 150
calories
    counting "rules," 189–90
    restricting, 15–16, 192–93
    of saturated fats, 17
CalorieKing website, 175
Caper-Dijon Vinaigrette, for Tuna Niçoise, 146, *147*
Caramelized 3-Onion Dip, *156*, 157
carbohydrates. *See also* sucrose
    avoiding at night, 186
    for breakfast, 55
    fiber, 54
    high-protein, low-carb diet study, 194
    metabolism of, 57
    restricted in diet study, 192
carrots
    Bison Hanger Steak with Chimichurri and Grilled Carrots, 90, *91*
    Buffalo Legs, 154
    Thai(riffic) Salmon Salad with Peanut-Lime Vinaigrette, 150
Cashews, with Superfast Chicken, *118*, 119
cauliflower
    Chicken Tikka Masala with Roasted Cauliflower, 94
    Curried Cauliflower Soup, 127
    Roasted Veg Buddha Bowl with Tahini Dressing, 138
Centers for Disease Control, diet and health study, 10
Cheese and Snackers, 166
chicken
    BBQ Chicken Coleslaw, 125
    Buffalo Chicken Wedge with Buffalo Ranch Dressing, 126
    Chicken Oreganata, *92*, 93
    Chicken Tikka Masala with Roasted Cauliflower, 94, *95*
    Five-Spice Seared Salmon with Mu Shu Vegetables, 85

Greek God Salad with Red Wine Vinaigrette, 128

Grilled Chicken Enchilada with Summer Squash and Chili Roja, 98, *99*

Killer Kale Salad with Roasted Garlic Vinaigrette, 131

lean meat and protein, 56–57

Pastaless Grilled-Vegetable Primavera Salad with Creamy Italian Dressing, 132

Santa Fe Chopped Salad with Smoky Ranch Dressing, 137

Semi-Caesar Salad, 140

Semisweet & Sour Chicken Salad with White Truffle Soy vinaigrette, *112*, 113

Spinach–Grilled Chicken Superfast Chicken & Cashews, *118*, 119

Chicken Oreganata, *92*, 93

Chicken Tikka Masala with Roasted Cauliflower, 94, *95*

Chili Roja, 98

Chili, Smoke-Signal Buffalo, 116

China Study, The, 25

chocolate, Dark Bark, *160*, 161

cholesterol
chemicals and effects on, 185
diets and lowering of, 24
exercise and effects on, 180
Friedewald equation, 30
high-density liopoproteins (HDL), 30–35
insulin and, 14
intermittent fasting, 192
low-carb, low-fat diets and, 15
low-density lipoproteins (LDL), 30–33, *34*, 35
maintaining healthy level, 191
medication for, versus diet and exercise, 6–7, 24
reducing, with Man Diet, 22, 24
tests, improved, 29–35
triglycerides, 17, 26, 29, 30, 32–34, 50, 56, 182
very low-density lipoprotein (VLDL), 14, 33, *34*
Weight Watchers and, 25

chromium, 51

chylomicrons, 32–33

coleslaw, BBQ Chicken, 125

Cocoa–Mixed Nut Energy Bars, 158, *159*

Columbia University study on technology and weight loss, 175

Copenhagen City Heart Study, 33

Cordain, Dr. Loren, 25

Cornell University study of shopping while hungry, 178

cortisol, 46, 48–51, 184

Creamy Italian Dressing, for Pastaless Grilled-Vegetable Primavera Salad, 132, *133*

Creole Tofu-Vegetable Étoufée, *96*, 97

Cucumber-Dill Sauce, for Turkey Jerky Kabobs, 117

Curried Cauliflower Soup, 127

Cushing's disease, 48

D

D'Adamo, Peter J., 25

Dark Bark, *160*, 161

Devilish Eggs, 162, *163*

diabetes
body muscle mass and, 182
fruit and effects on, 10
glycated hemoglobin and fasting insulin levels, 35–37
HbA1c test, 35–37
type 2, 14, 35
whole grains and reduced risk, 15

Diabetes Prevention Program, 165

dieting. *See also names of individual diets*
cheating, intelligently, 178–80
with family and/or friends, 175

dips. *See also dressings; sauces; vinaigrettes*
Brocc-amole with Jicama, 153
Caramelized 3-Onion Dip, *156*, 157
Gav-Spacho, 134

"Dirty Dozen" list of pesticide-affected produce, 61–62

di-2-ethylhexyl phthalate (DEHP), 185

dressings. *See also dips; sauces; vinaigrettes*
Avocado-Wasabi Dressing, for Baja Cobb Salad, 123
for BBQ Chicken Coleslaw, 125
Buffalo Ranch Dressing, for Buffalo Chicken Wedge, 126
Caesar, for Semi-Caesar Salad, 140, *141*
Caper-Dijon Vinaigrette, for Tuna Niçoise, 146, *147*
Creamy Italian Dressing, for Pastaless Grilled-Vegetable Primavera, 132, *133*
Honey Mustard Vinaigrette, for Sous Chef Salad, 138
horseradish, for Philly Cheesesteak Salad, 135
One Hundred–Island Dressing, for Turkey Burger Tostado, 148, *149*
Peanut-Lime Vinaigrette, for Thai(riffic) Salmon Salad, 150
Pesto Vinaigrette, for Summer Garden Salad, 144, *145*
Red Wine Vinaigrette, for Greek God Salad, 128, *129*
Roasted Garlic Vinaigrette, with Killer Kale Salad, *130*, 131
Smoky Ranch Dressing, for Santa Fe Chopped Salad, 137
Tahini Dressing, for Roasted Veg Buddha Bowl, 138
White Truffle Soy Vinaigrette, for Spinach–Grilled Chicken Salad, *142*, 143

Duke University study (STRRIDE) of exercise, 182

E

eating slowly versus quickly, 179

eating out, 177

Eat Right for Your Type, 25

Eco-Atkins diet, 27

eggs, 71, 89, 123, 139, 150
(Are You Kiddin' Me!) Crustless Quiche, 66, *67*
Basic Baked Eggs, *70*, 71
Devilish Eggs, 162, *163*
Fast Track Frittata, 72, *73*
Huevos Rancheros, 69
Micro Scramble, 68
1-2-3 Scramble, 68

Salmon "Steak" and Eggs with Asparagus and Lemon-Dill Yogurt Sauce, 80, *81*

Environmental Working Group and "Dirty Dozen" list, 61–62

European Heart Journal, 183

European Congress of Endocrinology, 41

exercise
aerobic, 181, 182
cholesterol, effects on, 180
FITT (frequency, intensity, type, time), 180–83
frequency of, 181
heart rate calculation, 181
high-intensity interval training, 181–82
personal digital assistant, 175
resting metabolic rate (RMR) and, 190
Studies of a Targeted Risk Reduction Intervention through Defined Exercise (STRRIDE), 182
time spent on, 183
types of, 182
walking, 181
weight training, 182

F

fast food restaurant study, 177

fasting glucose level, 23

fasting, intermittent, 192

Fast Track Frittata, 72, *73*

fat
body, measurement of, 39–40
psychological vulnerability and, 49

fats
mono- and polyunsaturated, 18
saturated, 17–19

fiber
All-Bran Buds, 54, 55, 76
Get Up & Go Granola, 76, *77*
SmartBran, 54, 55, 76
soluble, 56
versus starch, 9–10

fish and seafood, 58
Five-Spice Seared Salmon with Mu Shu Vegetables, *84*, 85
Salmon "Steak" and Eggs with Asparagus and Lemon-Dill Yogurt Sauce, 80
Sangria Salmon, 110, *111*
Thai(riffic) Salmon Salad with Peanut-Lime Vinaigrette, 150
Walnut-Sage Crusted Trout with Green Beans, 120, *121*

FITT (frequency, intensity, type, time) prescription for exercise, 180

Five-Spice Seared Salmon with Mu Shu Vegetables, *84*, 85

food labels
Multi Grain Cheerios, *55*
and study of restaurants, 177
Twinkie, *11*

food pyramid, 13

Forks over Knives, 25

Fresh Start Salad, *74*, 75

Friedewald equation, 30

Fritatta, Fast-Track, 72, *73*

fructose versus sucrose, 10

fruit. *See also berries*

Roasted Pear with Cinnamon Ricotta and Toasted Almonds, 168, *169*
smoothies, 10

G

Gav-Spacho, 134
genes versus lifestyle, 187
Get Up & Go Granola, 76, *77*
ghrelin
    effects on appetite, 179–80, 195–96
    effects on sleep, 185
glucagon, 50
gluten-free diets, 26–27
glycated hemoglobin (HbA1c) test, 19, 35
glycemic index, 14
Granola, Get Up and Go, 76
Greek God Salad with Red Wine Vinaigrette, 128, *129*
Greek yogurt, 79
Greenwich Hospital, 20
Grilled Carrots, with Bison Hanger Steak with Chimichurri, 90
Grilled Chicken Enchilada with Summer Squash and Chili Roja, 98, *99*
Green Beans, with Walnut-Sage Crusted Trout, 120, *121*
Grilled Sweet Chili Pork Tenderloin with Asparagus, *100*, 101
guacamole variation, Brocc-amole with Jicama, 152, 153
gut flora, 186–88

H

Halton, Thomas, 57
Harvard study of fast food restaurants, 177
Harvard T.H. Chan School of Public Health, 14
Harvard University's Department of Nutrition, 57
Harvard University's School of Public Health, 10
Hashimoto's thyroiditis, 45
health coaches, 175
heart attack risk, lowering, 185
heart disease
    cardiac CRP test, 37–38
    and diabetes, San Antonio study, 8
    homocysteine levels, 37–38
heart rate calculation, 181
heart muscle
    affected by cortisol, 49
    marathon runners and, 183
Honey Mustard Vinaigrette, for Sous Chef Salad, 138
Hoppin' Joe, 102, *103*
hormones
    effects on appetite, 179–80
    melatonin and sleep, 184
Horsey Sauce, for Philly Cheesesteak Salad, 135
Huevos Rancheros, 69
Hu, Frank, 57
homocysteine levels, 37–38

I

inflammation, 33, 37–38, 56
insulin, 13–14. *See also* blood glucose; cholesterol
    fasting levels, and glycated hemoglobin, 35–37
    levels, 185
    resistance, 14, 37, 50–51, 185, 92
International Expert Committee, 36
International Journal of Obesity, 184

J

Journal of the American College of Cardiology, 30, 38, 49
Journal of the American College of Nutrition, 57
Journal of the American Medical Association, 177, 186, 193

K

Kabat-Zinn, John, 188–89
ketone bodies, 16
Killer Kale Salad with Roasted Garlic Vinaigrette, *130*, 131

L

Lancet, The
    research on mummies, regarding Paleo diet, 26
    study of saturated fat effects, 18
LDL particle number, 29–35
lean meat/protein, 12, 56–57
Lemon-Dill Yogurt Sauce, with Salmon "Steak" and Eggs with Asparagus, 80
leptin
    effects on appetite, 179–80, 195–96
    effects on sleep, 185
lifestyle versus genes, 187
LoseIt! application, 176
low-carbohydrate, high protein diets, 16, 23, 24, 26, 194
low glycemic foods, 191
low-starch, -sucrose, and -saturated fat, 20–21
lunch and dinner, of Man Diet, 56–60

M

Man Diet
    Greenwich Hospital study of, 20–23
    summary, 53
Man Up Blueberry-Almond Muffins, *164*, 165
marinades
    Sweet Chili, for Grilled Pork Tenderloin, for Chicken Tikka Masala, 94
MB-EAT, 188–89
meals
    ready-made, 178
    restaurant, study of, 177
    structured, 88
Meatballs, Oven-Roasted, with Vegetable Caponata, *104*, 105
medications for weight loss, 50–51
Mediterranean diet, 23–24, 62–63, 192
MESA study, 38

metabolic syndrome
    described, 6
    diabetes and, 8
    exercise, and effects on, 180–82
    Man Diet and, 23
    nuts, and reversal of, 50
    resting metabolic rate (RMR), 190
    salt and, 51
    STRRIDE study, 185
    testosterone and, 40–41
    tests for, 31
metabolism, effects of hormones on, 41
Micro Scramble, 68
milks, kinds of, 56
mindfulness-based eating (MB-EAT), 188–89
mousse, Raspberry-Almond, 167
Muffins, Man Up Blueberry-Almond, *164*, 165
Multi-Ethnic Study of Atherosclerosis (MESA), The, 31, 38
Multi Grain Cheerios, 54–55
Mu-Shu Vegetables, with Five-Spice Seared Salmon, 85
muscle mass versus fat, 39, 40, 182, 193–94
MyFitnessPal, 176
MyPlate, 176

N

National College Institute, 41
National Health and Nutrition Examination Survey (NHANES) 2003–2006 population study, 36, 37, 38, 44, 47, 182
National Institute of Diabetes and Digestive and Kidney Diseases, 189
National Institutes of Health, 186
neuropeptides, and appetite control, 185
New England Journal of Medicine, 14, 15, 19, 23, 24, 29, 187 195
NHANES studies, 36, 37, 38, 44, 47, 182
NMR LipoProfile, 30
nonstick pans and effect on cholesterol, 185
nut oils, 50
nuts
    Almonds, Toasted, and Roasted Pear with Cinnamon Ricotta, 168, *169*
    Cashews, with Superfast Chicken, *118*, 119
    Cocoa–Mixed Nut Energy Bars, 158, *159*
    Get Up & Go Granola, 76
    and metabolic syndrome, 62
    Walnut-Sage Crusted Trout with Green Beans, 120

O

oatmeal, 55
obesity
    body mass index (BMI) measurement of, 39
    diabetes risk and, San Antonio study, 8
    effects of hormones, 41
    effect of plastic and packing pollutants, 185
    international conference, 39
    International Journal of Obesity and study of sleep, 184
    leptin and, 179
    lifestyle, sedentary, 13
    myths and facts, 187–88

pesticides as cause of, 61
stress and, 49
waist-to-height (WHtR) measurement of,
39–40
One Hundred–Island Dressing, for Turkey
Burger Tostado, 148, *149*
omega-3 fatty acids, 56, 62
one-pot meals
(Are You Kiddin' Me!) Crustless Quiche, 66
Hoppin' Joe, 102, *103*
Smoke Signal Buffalo Chili, 116
1-2-3 Scramble, 68
Open Heart study on saturated fat, 18
Ornish, Dean, 18
Ornish diet, 18–19
Oven-Roasted Meatballs with Vegetable
Caponata, *104*, 105

P
Paleo Diet, 12, 25, 26
Pan-Seared Beef Tenderloin with Shiitakes,
Lemon and Parsley, 106, *107*
Pastaless Grilled-Vegetable Primavera Salad
with Creamy Italian Dressing, 132, *133*
Peanut-Lime Vinaigrette, for Thai(riffic)
Salmon Salad, 150
Pear, Roasted, with Cinnamon Ricotta and
Toasted Almonds, 168, *169*
personal digital assistant, 175
Pesto Vinaigrette, for Summer Garden Salad,
144, *145*
Philly Cheesesteak Salad with Horsey Sauce,
135
Pinto Bean Stew, with Ancho Pork, 88, 89
plateau phase of weight loss, 189–190
pork
Allspice-Rubbed Pork Tenderloin with
Braised Red Cabbage and Grain Mustard,
86, *87*
Ancho Pork and Pinto Bean Stew, *88*, 89
Braised Low-Country Pork Chops, 83
Grilled Sweet Chili Pork Tenderloin with
Asparagus, *100*, 101
portabella mushrooms
Pastaless Grilled-Vegetable Primavera
Salad, 132
Sloppy (Doctor) Joes, 114, *115*
poultry, 56–57
preparing food in advance, 176
protein. *See also* Atkins diet
keeping weight off, 195
increasing amounts of, 193–94
lean, 12, 53, 56–57
too much, 194
pulses (beans), 58–59
Ancho Pork and Pinto Bean Stew, *88*, 89
(Are You Kiddin' Me!) Crustless Quiche,
66, *67*
BBQ Chicken Coleslaw, *124*, 125
Devilish Eggs, 162, *163*
Huevos Rancheros, 69
Ornish diet and, 18
Santa Fe Chopped Salad with Smoky
Ranch Dressing, *136*, 137
South of the Border 7-Layer Parfait, *170*,
171

Q
quiche, 66, *67*

R
Rainbow Beef Stir-Fry, *108*, 109
Raspberry-Almond Mousse, 167
Red, White and Blueberry Yogi Bowl, *78*, 79
Red Wine Vinaigrette, for Greek God Salad,
128, *129*
restaurants, and study of food labels, 177
resting metabolic rate (RMR), 190
rewards, to keep weight off, 195
Roasted Cauliflower, with Chicken Tikka
Masala, 94, *95*
Roasted Garlic Vinaigrette, with Killer Kale
Salad, *130*, 131
Roasted Pear with Cinnamon Ricotta and
Toasted Almonds, 168, *169*
Roasted Veg Buddha Bowl with Tahini
Dressing, 138
Roberts, Susan, 177

S
salad
Baja Cobb Salad with Avocado-Wasabi
Dressing, 123
BBQ Chicken Coleslaw, 125
Buffalo Chicken Wedge with Buffalo
Ranch Dressing, 126
Fresh Start Salad, *74*, 75
Gav-Spacho, 134
Greek God Salad with Red Wine
Vinaigrette, 128, *129*
Killer Kale Salad with Roasted Garlic
Vinaigrette, *130*, 131
Santa Fe Chopped Salad with Smoky
Ranch Dressing, 137
Semi-Caesar Salad, 140, *141*
Sous Chef Salad with Honey Mustard
Vinaigrette, 138
Spinach–Grilled Chicken Salad with White
Truffle Soy Vinaigrette, *142*, 143
Summer Garden Salad with Pesto
Vinaigrette, 144, *145*
Thai(riffic) Salmon Salad with Peanut-Lime
Vinaigrette, 150
Tuna Niçoise with Caper-Dijon Vinaigrette,
146, *147*
Turkey Burger Tostado with One Hundred–
Island Dressing, 148, *149*
salmon
Five-Spice Seared Salmon with Mu Shu
Vegetables, *84*, 85
Salmon "Steak" and Eggs with Asparagus
and Lemon-Dill Yogurt Sauce, 80, *81*
Sangria Salmon, 110, *111*
Thai(riffic) Salmon Salad with Peanut-Lime
Vinaigrette, 150
salt
cortisol levels and 49–50
and metabolic syndrome, 50
San Antonio Breast Cancer Symposium, 192
Sangria Salmon, 110, *111*
Santa Fe Chopped Salad with Smoky Ranch
Dressing, *136*, 137

saturated fats, 17–19
sauces. *See also* dips; dressings; vinaigrettes
Chili Roja, for Grilled Chicken Enchilada
with Summer Squash, 98, *99*
Chimichurra, for Bison Hanger Steak and
Grilled Carrots, 90, *91*
Cucumber-Dill Sauce, for Turkey Jerky
Kabobs, 117
Horsey Sauce, for Philly Cheesesteak
Salad, 135
Lemon-Dill Yogurt Sauce, for Salmon
"Steak" and Eggs with Asparagus, 80
Sangria, for Salmon, 110, *111*
semisweet, for Semisweet & Sour Chicken,
112, 113
for Superfast Chicken & Cashews, 119
tomato, for Sloppy (Doctor) Joes, 114, *115*
Science, 193
self-acceptance aspect of MB-EAT, 189
Semi-Caesar Salad, 140, *141*
Semisweet & Sour Chicken, *112*, 113
Shiitakes, with Pan-Seared Beef Tenderloin
with Lemon and Parsley, 106, *107*
shopping while hungry (Cornell University
study), 178
sleep, benefits of, 184–85
Sloppy (Doctor) Joes, 114, *115*
Smoke Signal Buffalo Chili, 116
Smoky Ranch Dressing, for Santa Fe Chopped
Salad, *136*, 137
Sous Chef Salad with Honey-Mustard
Vinaigrette, 139
South of the Border 7-Layer Parfait, *170*, 171
Spinach–Grilled Chicken Salad with White
Truffle Soy Vinaigrette, *142*, 143
Srikanthan, Dr. Preethi, 182
starch, 12–16, 19
steak
Grilled Carrots, with Bison Hanger Steak
with Chimichurri, 90, *91*
Pan-Seared Beef Tenderloin with Shiitakes,
Lemon and Parsley, 106, *107*
Philly Cheesesteak Salad with Horsey
Sauce, 135
Salmon "Steak" and Eggs with Asparagus
and Lemon-Dill Yogurt Sauce, 80, *81*
steroids, 48
stress
binge eating, 188
cortisol and weight gain, 48–51
sleep, and effect on weight loss, 184
management, and Ornish diet, 19
structured meals, 88
Studies of a Targeted Risk Reduction
Intervention through Defined Exercise,
(STRRIDE), 182
sucrose (table sugar), 9–11, 15
Summer Berry Fro-Yo Pops, 172, *173*
Summer Garden Salad with Pesto Vinaigrette,
144, *145*
Summer Squash and Chili Roja, with Grilled
Chicken Enchilada, 98, *99*
Superfast Chicken & Cashews, *118*, 119

T

Tahini Dressing, for Roasted Veg Buddha Bowl, 138
testosterone, 40–41
Thai(riffic) Salmon Salad with Peanut-Lime Vinaigrette, 150
thermogenic effect of protein, 194
thyroid
    antithyroperoxidase antibody (anti-TPO Ab), 45
    hypothyroidism, 44–46
    Hashimoto's thyroiditis, 45
    iodine deficiency, 46
    subclinical hypothyroidism, 42, 45–46
    thyroxine (T4) and triiodothyronine (T3), 46
    thyroid stimulating hormone (TSH), 42
    tests for, 45
tofu, in Creole Tofu-Vegetable Étoufée, 96, 97
triglycerides, 26, 29, 32–34, 50, 56, 182
Tufts University study of food labels, 177
Tuna Niçoise with Caper-Dijon Vinaigrette, 146, 147
turkey
    lean meat and poultry, 56–57
    Sloppy (Doctor) Joes, 114, 115
    Smoke Signal Buffalo Chili, 116
    Turkey Burger Tostada with One Hundred–Island Dressing, 148, 149
    Turkey Jerky Kabobs with Cucumber-Dill Sauce, 117
Turkey Burger Tostada with One Hundred–Island Dressing, 148, 149
Turkey Jerky Kabobs with Cucumber-Dill Sauce, 117
Twinkie label, 11

V

Vegetable Caponata, with Oven-Roasted Meatballs, 104, 105
vegetables. See also salads
    Braised Red Cabbage and Grain Mustard, with Five-Spice Rubbed Pork Tenderloin, 86, 87
    Brocc-amole with Jicama, 152, 153
    Creole Tofu-Vegetable Étoufée, 96, 97
    Grilled Carrots, with Bison Hanger Steak with Chimichurri, 90, 91
    Hoppin' Joe, 102, 103
    Mu Shu Vegetables, with Five-Spice Seared Salmon, 84, 85
    Pastaless Grilled-Vegetable Primavera Salad with Creamy Italian Dressing, 132, 133
    Rainbow Beef Stir-Fry, 108, 109
    Roasted Cauliflower, with Chicken Tikka Masala 94, 95
    Roasted Veg Buddha Bowl with Tahini Dressing, 138
    with Semisweet & Sour Chicken, 112, 113
    Vegetable Caponata, with Oven-Roasted Meatballs, 104, 105
vegetarianism, 18–19, 26, 58
vinaigrettes. See also dips; dressings; sauces

Caper-Dijon Vinaigrette, for Tuna Niçoise, 146, 147
Roasted Garlic Vinaigrette, for Killer Kale Salad, 131
White Truffle Soy Vinaigrette, for Semisweet & Sour Chicken Salad, 112, 113

W

waist-to-height (WHtR) measurement of fat, 39–40
walking, 181
Walnut-Sage Crusted Trout with Green Beans, 120, 121
weight loss drugs, 179, 186-88
weight training, Duke University study of, 182
Weight Watchers, 24–25
Weindruch, Dr. Richard, 193
White House Task Force on Obesity, 61
White Truffle Soy Vinaigrette, for Spinach–Grilled Chicken Salad, 142, 143
Women's Health Initiative, 58
Women's health
    San Antonio Breast Cancer Symposium, 192
    Women's Health Study (Harvard Univeristy), 183

Y

yogurt
    Lemon-Dill Yogurt Sauce, 80
    Red, White and Blueberry Yogi Bowl, 78, 79
    South of the Border 7-Layer Parfait, 170, 171
    Summer Berry Fro-Yo Pops, 172, 173